LONDON FORD

Ladyish

First edition

ISBN: 9798359134064

This book was professionally typeset on Reedsy.
Find out more at reedsy.com

Contents

Introduction

You *define beauty yourself. Society doesn't define your beauty.* - Lady Gaga

Lady Gaga is absolutely right.

Beauty has nothing to do with those around you; it is how you see yourself.

Believing in your beauty is easier said than done. I know this firsthand.

Growing up is hard. It can feel awkward. It's frustrating. I remember standing in front of my bathroom mirror wondering, "When am I going to look grown up?" I'd pinch my stomach and thighs just hoping that, someday, I'd look like the models I saw on billboards and in magazines.

For a while, I walked through life feeling jealous. I looked chill on the outside; on the inside, I felt anything but.

We live in a world surrounded by comparisons and it's damaging to your confidence. Confidence might be key, but you have to find the lock you fit into before opening the door.

This book is your lock.

You're probably feeling a cluster of emotions right now. Being a teenager is complicated: You have school (math class is kicking your butt), activities, extracurriculars (maybe your parents encouraged you to join key club or the honors society), friendships, partners, etc. — the whole nine yards.

It's a lot to handle, and on top of that, your body is changing in ways you don't quite understand.

Not too long ago, I was in your shoes. I'm here to help.

This book is a sequel to the book, *Girlish*, which discussed the changes inside your growing body. *Girlish* focuses on the changes and feelings you have while entering puberty, but now you're more grown up, and puberty (and what comes after) is right in front of you.

Many topics surrounding puberty, sexuality, confidence, and your changing emotions are often kept quiet. These are the topics that make for awkward living room conversations with parents and sniggering classroom lessons. So many people never find all the information you need to understand your body and how to enter adulthood.

These topics are important. They're crucial. You deserve to know what's happening and how to cope, and I've done the work for you.

I've spent my career helping teens and young girls understand their bodies to prepare them for a happy, healthy life. Myths and confusions are everywhere, but they're just that — myths. I want to help you understand the process from start to finish so you can avoid the awkward and uncomfortable conversations I went through.

This book will discuss the ins and outs of being a teen. We'll cover the following topics.

- periods and how to cope with them
- changes in thoughts and mood
- the value of a good night's sleep
- how to fuel your body

2

- bras, healthy sex, and sexuality
- gender norms and expression
- body positivity

Think about your life five years from now. Do you want to go to college or get a job? Do you want to feel more confident or feel more positive about yourself and what you can do? Would you like to feel more educated about your sexuality and expression?

Probably.

Growing up isn't easy — it takes time and practice. I spent most of my young adult life in the dark because I didn't know where to begin.

It doesn't have to be that way. To accomplish your goals, you need to know all the info.

You can't just talk the talk, you need to walk the walk.

I ask you to reflect while you read. You deserve a life worth dreaming about.

Chapter 1: Celebrating the New You

So, you've had your first period. Maybe you've had a few (or more than a few) by now. You've experienced the cramps, the moodiness, and maybe even some bloating. How do you feel? Many girls feel confused, upset, or maybe even angry. Hopefully, you feel a little excited. I remember jumping for joy and running to tell my mother when I got my first period.

Many girls find periods to be frustrating, time-consuming, embarrassing, and annoying. But they don't have to be that way. There's nothing to be embarrassed by.

Most girls and women experience periods; we're all in the same boat.

Periods don't have to be a depressing reality. They're meant to be positive! They're a sign that your body is right on track. You're becoming an adult! You're changing. Well, scratch that. You're *evolving*. Periods are a huge part of growing up and becoming a strong, powerful baddie.

It's okay to feel a little ashamed; everything you are feeling is perfectly normal! Talking about your body and what's happening isn't taboo. Let's talk about some things you can expect when getting your period.

Period Lingo: When It Starts and The Aftermath

Most women start their period around two years after the onset of puberty, usually between the ages of ten and sixteen. That's a pretty wide window, and anything in between is perfectly normal. If you're a little earlier or a little later, that's okay too! It's *your* body first, and normal can mean many different things.

There are a wide variety of factors that influence the onset of your first period, including: diet, exercise routine, family history, or even your environment (Behring, 2019). You can't control these factors, so don't worry if you're a little behind or ahead of the curve. As I said, it's your body, and listening to it is important.

So how can you prepare?

You may be nervous or even embarrassed, but preparing for and tracking your periods helps minimize these feelings. Think about this example: when you have a test at school, you likely feel less anxious if you study and bring sharpened pencils, right?

Right.

Carrying period products, like tampons and pads, and having them accessible can help you minimize this stress. When I began my period, I was worried about it starting in the middle of the school day — and it did a few times. So I carried around a pencil case with tampons, a stress ball, and a few pads, so I'd be prepared.

Getting your first period is stressful, but many girls find that the few periods after this are just as stressful and nerve-wracking.

Your period may be irregular for a while, and that is, again, perfectly normal. There could be months where you don't have one at all, and that's to be expected. Think about what your body is going through. It hasn't experienced this reaction either. It takes time to get used to new things. When you first started riding a bike, you probably fell off a few times before you got good at it. Your body works the same way.

Listen to your body. It's pretty good at communicating.

Let's dive into what you can expect when starting your periods.

What to Expect From PMS

Premenstrual Syndrome, otherwise known as PMS, affects nearly 80% of women and girls experiencing their period. That sounds a little scary. Think about it this way: you're in the same boat as 80% of the women around you. There's strength in numbers. You're not alone.

PMS sounds scary. When you begin your period, that's likely one of the first things you're afraid of. Movies and media don't make it any easier. Google doesn't help at all. So what can you *really* expect when experiencing PMS?

PMS is a period where hormonal interactions in your body trigger the release of the uterine lining. Estrogen, androgen, and other hormones with long, science-y names all play a role. Muscles and organs get involved and they all work together to shed the lining because you're not pregnant.

Honestly, it's a lot of work. Your body is really grinding to get it all out.

But what do you experience? All that work has to come with certain effects, right?

Many women report feeling moody, tired, and a little irritable before starting their cycle. Some women listen to Taylor Swift or Olivia Rodrigo and cry a little. You might feel more angry than normal or forget to bring a black pen to class. The emotional symptoms are scary, and though they aren't exactly a good time, there are many ways we can learn to deal with them and accept them. We'll cover this in the next section.

Some women experience more physical symptoms like increases or changes in appetite, lower back pain, and breakouts. You might find yourself reaching for the chocolate bar on the top shelf of your kitchen cabinet. You might ask your mom or another family member to borrow their heating pad or find a few little whiteheads on your chin. It's to be expected.

I'm not telling you this to scare you. You shouldn't feel scared at all! In fact, anxiety and worry can make a lot of these symptoms worse. Being prepared and knowing how to work through it is important. Just like the studying example, you'll feel more confident if you can combat it.

Takin' Care of Business: The Guide to Managing PMS

So like... how do I manage it? It's not like you can study for it or bring a notebook. Preparedness is key to managing your PMS symptoms and to becoming your own period girl boss.

Think about the symptoms you've experienced and the ones above. How might you go about managing those using the tools you already have? Before you reach for your parent's Midol bottle, let's talk about some other skills and habits you can try. I'll give you some pointers.

Managing Your Crazy Moods

You're a mood-swing kinda gal. Guess what, me too. Before my period, I get a little cranky. I cry during sad movies, and I feel much more anxious than normal. It sucks — but I plan.

If you feel you might be one of those people (most period-peeps are), think about what you can do to manage your symptoms. It begins with you.

Try taking care of yourself. Use self-care. Self-care gets a bad rep. It doesn't necessarily involve pouring your heart and soul into a little pink journal, nor does it have to involve a relaxing bubble bath. Of course, if those sound appealing, try them out!

Think about what you do during your free time right now. Do you play sports or enjoy jogging? Maybe you like to read, dance, or play certain video games.

Why do you like those activities? Do you feel a sense of accomplishment after finishing a challenging race? Do you feel energized after rehearsal? Maybe reading calms you down and brings you into a whole different world. Start there. You can't be expected to abandon your entire routine just for a few days. Think about the habits you currently enjoy and use them as tools to manage your symptoms. Oftentimes, distraction is the name of the game.

If you find you've lost interest in some of those activities during your pre-period, that's also okay, and quite common. A lot of women experience a loss of interest in things they normally enjoy during this time. If you feel that applies to you, that doesn't mean you should throw in the towel.

Try something new, even if it's as simple as taking a few hours to binge-watch your favorite show on Netflix. The possibilities are endless.

Here are some things you can try if you feel like nothing else works.

- Go for a walk. If you have a dog or a friend who'd like to tag along, bring them. You don't have to do this alone. If not, try walking by yourself in a place you feel safe. Go during the daytime and take in what's around you. At the very least, you'll occupy yourself for a little while.
- Listen to music. Any music will do. If you're an alternative gal, try checking out some new free music on YouTube or Spotify. If you like Pop, try listening to the radio. Whatever floats your boat.
- Phone a friend or family member. As I said, 80% of women and girls are in the exact same boat. They might not have their period at the same time as you, but it's likely you know other people who have walked in your shoes. Talk it out. Your mother, female guardian, sibling, friend, or trusted counselor or teacher has been where you are right now. They might even have some insight into other things you can do and try.
- Avoid stressful situations. That doesn't mean you can't submit your homework or take tests, but avoid the stressful situations you can control. This isn't the time to ask your crush on a date. That can wait until next week. Focus on what you need to do to make yourself feel better.
- Take time for yourself. Sometimes we need a breather. It's okay to be alone sometimes. While you're taking your break, take the time to think about what you're feeling. Be mindful of what's going on in your head. Anything you feel is okay.

If you have concerns about what's going on, talk to someone: a family member, guardian, friend, teacher, counselor, medical professional, or other resource. If you feel what you're experiencing is abnormal, be your own advocate!

Confronting the Physical

The physical symptoms of PMS can be scary, but, like I said, preparation is key. Listen to your body. If you find yourself craving chocolate and other sweets, try to prepare for that. Ask a parent or guardian to buy an extra bar of chocolate at the grocery store, or pick up your favorite candy at the bodega down the street. Be safe about it, and don't binge eat, but take the steps you feel you need to make yourself feel comfy.

Some women and period girlies experience bloating or weight gain. Don't freak out! It's temporary. Again, the hormones in your body are doing a lot of work, and this can cause things to go out of whack for a bit. Unfortunately, I fall into this boat too. It's okay to worry a bit, but manage your worries. Remember, it's not real, and it's not something out of the ordinary.

Try not to weigh yourself during your period week. Again, it doesn't matter, your weight will be back to normal in no time. Try to fuel your body with snacks you find healthy and delicious. Treat yourself. It's okay to feel a little discouraged, but being aware is important. Rationalize what's happening. You aren't alone.

If you find yourself breaking out more than normal during your pre-period, that's okay! Again, I relate. I used to fret and grow anxious and pop pimples erratically, but this didn't help. I was still breaking out and then my skin was just red. We have to prepare for it. Keep up with your normal skincare routine and remember that this is *temporary*. It will go away as soon as your period is over. Pimples are scary and stubborn, so don't work yourself up. Stress will only make it worse.

Keep doing what you normally do. Maybe purchase a few inexpensive face masks to use during your pre-period. Try a steaming technique or do a DIY mask (egg whites or honey are both quite effective). Stay safe, but branch out a bit. Taking the extra time to care for your skin will make you feel 100% better.

Maybe you experience cramping or lower back pain. Don't be alarmed. It's normal too. Instead of popping Advil, focus on mindfully acknowledging the symptoms. Take a rest or go to bed early. Use a heating pad or ask someone you trust to give you a mini-massage. It's not comfortable, but it's not supposed to be. You're a growing adult.

Getting your period is part of adulting. It's your first big girl experience. Big girls take charge of their feelings and manage them. They know what they need to do and take care of business. Be your own big girl and don't be afraid to ask for help. Big girls, even the best ones, need a little push sometimes.

You aren't alone. You're growing.

Cultural Traditions and Celebrations

In many cultures, getting your period involves tradition and celebration. You're becoming a woman, after all! This is what you've been waiting for! Let's take a look at some of the cultural traditions surrounding menstruation. Your findings might surprise you.

Traditions in Brazil and Columbia

The Tikuna tribe of South America celebrates a woman's first menstruation in what's called the Pelazon tradition. The Pelazon tradition is a time of empowerment; when young Tikuna women experience their first period, they're sent to live in a special, private room in their family's home for up to one whole year. During this time, they're allowed one special visitor, usually a grandmother, who teaches the young Tikuna women weaving, medicine, special tribe traditions, and the importance of family (Aquino, 2020).

The young woman learns her power as a woman and is allowed time to reflect on this important life experience. It's empowering.

After a year, the girl, now considered a woman, is led to the Maloka, where the tribe holds its most sacred ceremonies. The woman is covered in a rich blue pigment called uito and the tribe celebrates her newfound womanhood for three whole days.

The Tikuna tribe celebrates her feminine individuality as something to be proud of, not ashamed of. After all, your period is among the first signs that you're ready to be a woman.

It's a beautiful thing!

Ojibwe Celebrations

The Tikuna tribe isn't the only one that uses isolation periods to celebrate womanhood. The Ojibwe tribe of the North American Midwest celebrates menstruation through a period of careful reflection. Menstruating Ojibwe women spend time with others going through the process in what they call a moon lodge (Aquino, 2020). They're given a break from normal tasks and use this peaceful time to embrace the changes happening in their bodies.

This practice strengthens the female bond in the Ojibwe community and provides growing women with the space to experience the joys of womanhood.

West African Traditions

In areas of West Africa, namely Ghana, they celebrate menstruating women like goddesses. When a woman begins her first period, she's placed under a large, peaceful umbrella; members of her family and the surrounding community present her with food, gifts, and support (Brink, 2015). Her adulthood is lauded and appreciated by her community, and she's made to feel safe and comfortable through her exciting transition.

What about me?

It's unlikely your parents or guardians will let you spend a year in your room to celebrate your growth, but there are small things you can do to embrace the changes happening in your beautiful body.

Consider the Tikuna traditions; ask those around you about their experiences with womanhood and use their advice to guide your growth. Take time to reflect and develop new skills and personal traditions. Treat yourself like the women in West Africa. Many women, including myself, habitually buy a chocolate or candy bar before their period.

Celebrate in little ways. You deserve it.

Collaborate and communicate with the women around you.

The Ojibwe tradition of celebrating among other women is something you can practice. Talk to your friends about their experiences and lean on those around you. Everyone's going through the same thing, right? We don't have to do it alone. Support each other as you grow into this new phase of your life.

Celebrate The Positives

It's not all chocolate, heating pads, and sad songs. Your period is a sign that you're entering a new and exciting phase of your life. You're stepping into womanhood in very cute shoes. This is the part of your life where you make the decisions. You're in control. Adulting involves a lot of freedom. Embrace it. Love it. Be it.

You may not yet realize it, but having your period is a very good thing. Let's talk about the benefits of getting your period.

Periods Help You Work Out Harder

You read that right. Bear with me: The hormones that trigger your period actually improve your body's physical endurance. During your period, your progesterone levels drop, which gives your body access to the energy it needs to fight activity burnout. You become more focused and powerful (Jones, 2016).

I know what you're thinking, "The last thing I wanna do is go to the gym." I get it — motivation is tough when you feel pre-period fatigue. This is the time to get empowered. Take advantage of that energy and use it to your advantage.

Not only that, but working out can lessen that achy, cranky feeling you get during this time. Exercise can help shorten your periods and make them less heavy.

You've probably heard of "runner's high," or the happy, accomplished, energized feeling you get after intense physical activity. If you're experiencing depressed moods or moodiness in general, exercising can help minimize those feelings and provide you with a sense of worthwhile satisfaction.

Periods Can Slow Aging

Yup. Adulthood is exciting, but let's face it. No one *wants* to get old. Luckily, periods are likely one of the causes of increased life expectancy among women.

It's science. Iron, a mineral present in your blood, releases every month during your period. While iron does a lot of great things for the body, it can also contribute to free radical production, which isn't so cool (Jones, 2016). Excess free radicals can cause age-related diseases and unnecessary oxidative stress to your cells.

So the next time you feel ashamed of your period or jealous of your male counterparts, remember this: your period is causing you to live longer. Kind of a flex, right?

Periods Keep You In-Tune with your Health

Periods are a woman's sort of signal. When something is wrong with your body, your period may become heavier or lighter. When it's late, that could be a sign that you're stressed or there's something wrong with your nutrient consumption.

Hormonal changes trigger periods. It's all in your thyroid. If your thyroid is functioning properly, your periods will be perfectly normal. If not, you'll likely see the signs pretty quickly.

Think of it as your body's personal traffic light. When your period is normal (whatever normal means for you), things are going as needed. You can move forward and follow the speed limit. If something is a bit off, that's the yellow light. You might need to think about stress or your diet. Proceed, but with caution. If your period is completely off, whether it's late or gone altogether, that's the red light. Stop and speak to a parent, guardian, nurse, or a trusted medical professional.

It's a Sign You're Not Pregnant

Your period is the most important sign you're not pregnant. Sometimes, it can be a huge relief. The uterine lining provides an embryo with nutrients; when you have your period, your body releases that lining because there's no embryo to nourish.

If you get your period, there's a low chance that you're pregnant.

It's an Excuse to Treat Yourself

We love to treat ourselves, or at least I do. Your period is the perfect excuse! Your body is putting in a lot of work; it's doing the most. Treat it like you would a friend who's going through a hard time.

Treating yourself doesn't necessarily mean spending a lot of money. There are many ways to treat yourself that don't involve money at all! You can binge-watch your favorite movie or TV show, or use it as an excuse to do a bit of reading.

Your period is the perfect time to take care of your body and to listen to its needs. Is it telling you to rest? Is it telling you it's hungry? Listen to it and give yourself a little extra lovin'.

Period Pennings

Your period is your body's way of telling you it's okay. There's nothing to fear. It's important to reflect on what you're experiencing. This is the time to think about you. You're a woman now. Celebrate!

Take some time to answer these questions. Writing them out is helpful, but you can answer them in your head too.

- _____has been on my mind this month. I think I feel _____way about it.
- _____, _____, and _____is what I've accomplished recently.
- I've been feeling _____during this cycle. I think I'll try _____ to manage it.
- I want to accomplish _____before my next cycle. I plan to start doing _____ and _____ to reach my goals.

Chapter 2: Sleepless Is My Middle Name

Are you a night owl or a morning person? Do you dream when you sleep or have nightmares? Do you often wake up?

All of that's normal. Setting positive sleep habits early in your life can prepare you for many restful nights in the future. Don't get me wrong, it's not easy. Staying up all night watching the latest season of *Outer Banks* or *The Bachelor* sounds fun and quite tempting, but the cranky, pounding feeling the morning after is anything but fun.

Think about how your sleep habits have changed over the last few years. Do you feel more sleepy during the day than you did as a child? There's certainly a reason for that.

Constant feelings of exhaustion stink. They really do. The groans and constant bags under your eyes aren't fun to deal with, and no amount of concealer can change how your fatigue negatively affects your daily activities.

So why are you so tired? How does puberty affect your sleep and, more importantly, how does sleep even work?

Let's explore!

So How Does Sleep Work?

Before we discuss the importance of sleep and tips to improve your sleep patterns, it's important to talk about how it works on a scientific level. Don't worry, it's anything but boring.

The Science of Sleep

Sleep is a nightly cycle. But luckily, it's not a complex one. Let's break it down.

There are four key stages of sleep you should be aware of.

Stage One: It lasts only for a few minutes (no more than five or ten). Your body knows it needs to sleep, so it has to get ready for the next steps. Unfortunately, this is the stage during which you're most likely to wake up.

Have you ever fallen asleep for a few seconds, only to be swiftly awoken by a siren outside or a loud noise? Yup, this is the stage where that happens.

Within just a few moments after finally closing your eyes, the body begins the process of sleep. Your heart rate and breathing slow and your body temperature drops. Don't panic, it's normal. A drop in these levels reduces the rate at which your body spends energy.

Stage Two: This stage is a bit longer and can last up to an hour. It's the preparation stage; your body is getting ready to enter deep sleep. You're less likely to be awoken during this stage, but it's just as important as any other. Your body's processes continue to slow down as less and less energy is used to maintain your bodily functions. The goal is to use this energy to heal your body in the next two stages.

Stage Three: This is the last stage your body experiences

19

prior to full REM (otherwise known as rapid eye movement) sleep. But we'll get into that later. This is the stage where you experience deep and restful sleep. You're not quite resting yet, but your muscles begin to relax and recharge from the previous day's activities.

In stage three, your body recharges your memory and critical thinking skills. That's why you might feel foggy after a restless night. We need time to recuperate and give our brains some rest. We deserve it!

Stage Four: This is the deepest stage of sleep, also known as REM sleep. You can think of it as the Dream Stage; your muscles and organs experience temporary paralysis (Suni, 2022). Again, don't be alarmed! It's perfectly normal. Think of it as the body's breather.

While your muscles are taking their rest, your brain activity increases and therefore, you dream. This stage is essential for brain growth and maintenance; we have to give our brain a rest, just like we would our body!

Beyond the Body: What Can't You Sleep?

As we get older, our sleep patterns change for a variety of reasons. Earlier, I asked you to consider how your sleep pattern has changed over the last few years. Maybe you've noticed a change much more recently, in the past few months. Perhaps you have noticed no changes at all. As we go through puberty, hormonal changes in our bodies affect when and how we sleep. It's natural and absolutely nothing to worry about. What you should understand is how it happens and how you can go about getting the best beauty sleep for you.

Hormonal Changes in Sleep

Puberty changes your circadian rhythm, or the 24-hour schedule your body naturally follows. A wide variety of factors, both environmental and hormonal affects your circadian rhythm. During puberty, your body's sleep clock shifts a few hours. Prior to puberty, the majority of children begin to feel sleepy around eight or nine PM. Following puberty, your body gets tired around ten or eleven PM (Better Health Channel, 2018).

This is called the "sleep phase delay." Our bodies are naturally programmed to need about eight hours of sleep per night (no matter what others may tell you), so instead of sleeping until five or six am, you might feel as though you need to sleep until eight or nine.

You're probably thinking, "There's no way I can sleep that late and still get to school on time!" Unfortunately, most school systems start classes much earlier than nine or ten am, making the two-hour adjustment in your body's sleep schedule more difficult to adapt to.

The Rise of Smartphones

We'll dive into the body's changes in sleep later in the section; let's first explore some of the other changes in your life that might affect your sleep schedule.

Most young teens use smart devices (laptops, phones, computers, etc.) to communicate with their friends and family in early puberty. Do you remember your excitement when you got your first smartphone? You were pretty stoked, right?

Social media is fun. YouTube videos are entertaining, and platforms like TikTok and Instagram make scrolling (and losing track of time) easy. I'm not saying you need to stay off social media. How boring would that be?

Instead, I want you to understand how social media and late-night scrolling affect your sleep cycle.

Unfortunately, the use of smartphones and laptops late at night can negatively affect your sleep schedule. According to sleep experts, teens who put up their smartphones an hour prior to going to bed get nearly a half hour of sleep more than their screen-glued counterparts (Better Health Channel, 2018).

School & Activity Schedules

Most teens hate waking up for school. I certainly did. I groaned in response to my alarm beeping every morning for years. It's okay, we all experience it. Very few teens consider themselves "morning people", and that's normal.

Beyond the mornings, your hectic after-school schedule can affect your sleep habits. Do you have volleyball practice, gymnastics, or theater rehearsal after school? Maybe you have a part-time job at your local coffee shop too. It's a lot to manage, especially when you have lots of homework or social engagements.

Let's explore.

Maybe your school day ends around 2:30 PM or three. You make your way to the dressing or locker room to change into your workout clothes or costumes before making your way to practice.

Practice is a few hours long (most activities rehearse for about two-three hours daily) and it's five or six PM before you know it! Your parent or guardian picks you up from practice and you rub your eyes. You're already a little tired (the coach is really pushing you this month).

You go home and eat dinner with your family, and realize it's already 7:30 PM! Crap. You have a chemistry exam on Friday, and you have to start studying. Not only that, but your English teacher loaded on a "surprise" essay due Saturday night. Maybe you have other small assignments to complete, too. You're overwhelmed. You grab a quick drink of water and sit in front of your laptop or computer for a few hours, pouring over PowerPoint and notes.

You barely notice the time tick-tocking away.

Before you know it, it's 11 PM, and you're still not in your jammies.

You get ready for bed and snuggle under the covers at 11:30. Your brain is stuffed. You're worried about your coach, and your exam grade, and wonder what you're going to wear tomorrow.

It's a lot. I know. Our increasingly crazy schedules only get crazier as we grow older. It stinks.

These activities cut into our sleep schedules and negatively affect how we feel throughout the day.

The Hustle

All of your activities compete for your time, and peer or parental pressure doesn't make it any easier. As we get older, we feel increased pressure to "hustle" or stay busy. Your part-time job, after-school clubs, and possible college application deadlines really keep you going throughout the day.

Unfortunately, it doesn't get much easier.

Pressure from friends and family can cause a great deal of stress. Maybe your mom wants you to start going to a new

23

club she heard about at school, or your guardian wants you to start ACT prep. The laundry list of extra activities seems never-ending. It's a lot to deal with!

The constant pressure to contribute more and more can affect your sleep habits. Activities and engagements pile on and soon, you're fully booked until 11 PM. After that, you stay awake a while and worry about what you have to do the next day. It's a lot. We have to remember the importance of sleep and how a lack of it can interfere with your ability to do what you've gotta do. We'll dive into that more later in the chapter, but for right now, consider how your activities and the "hustle" might be affecting your sleep habits.

You're Not Getting Enough Sleep. What Comes Next?

You're likely getting too little sleep. That's to be expected. You're a busy gal! So how does the hustle and lack of sleep affect your routine? What can happen if you're consistently low on sleep?

A lot.

Regularly receiving too little sleep can cause a lot of issues, including "cognitive defects, angry outbursts, negative mood, decreased attention, mental health issues, [and] learning issues" (Klein, 2019). Beyond the mental, a lack of sleep over a long period can cause serious physical ailments, including high blood pressure and obesity.

Doesn't sound fun, right?

Mental Effects

Lack of sleep consistently can cause serious mental health issues, including depression and anxiety. Additionally, some researchers note that too many sleepless nights can even cause suicidal behavior or ideation (Klein, 2019).

It's a cycle. A common symptom of depression is an increased desire to sleep. You might feel this a little already. When we feel bogged down by a never-ending list of to-dos, we become exhausted and lose interest in activities we previously loved. This makes us tired and depressed.

Your grades start to decline and your friends and family grow worried. Heck, maybe you're a little worried. It's hard feeling as though there's no way out of the cycle. It only gets worse. As certain tasks are neglected, they pile up. It seems like the list keeps getting longer.

It isn't easy, but sleeping and following a healthy sleep schedule can mitigate some symptoms of depression.

Anxiety is another side-effect of long-term sleeplessness. Again, it's a cycle. But one that we can stop in its tracks.

When we become anxious about tests, exams, activities, friends, jobs, and family, our sleep schedule falls by the wayside. You might find yourself up late at night worrying about what's coming the following day. Will you pass your science test? Will your crush finally like you back and will you remember your choreography at the final dance recital? It's stressful.

Staying up late worrying about it only hinders your ability to conquer your daily tasks. On average, those who maintain an adequate and healthy sleep schedule experience lessened symptoms of both depression and anxiety.

Physical Effects

But it's not just mental. Sleep is our body's time to recuperate and regroup. It's the breather our body needs to repair tissues and get us ready for the next day's challenges. Lack of sleep can cause obesity, high blood pressure, and developmental impairments.

The hormones released during sleep affect our ability to feel hunger or lack thereof. Again, it's science baby!

The hormone ghrelin is the hunger hormone, responsible for making us feel hungry throughout the day. On the other hand, the hormone leptin decreases hunger and provides a feeling of fullness (Pacheo, 2020). When we aren't sleeping well, the body increases ghrelin production and leptin levels decline. You feel hungrier more often and aren't able to regulate your food intake. This leads to weight gain, which can have dangerous long-term effects if not addressed.

While you sleep, your body processes slow down. Heart rate and blood pressure decrease to allow you to relax and rest. If you don't receive enough sleep, your blood pressure never gets the rest it desperately needs, causing higher blood pressure throughout the day. Unfortunately, this can lead to long-term issues, including heart disease and diabetes.

Sleep plays a role in your development. You're still growing and developing. You want your body to be the best it can be! In teens, certain hormones are released that aid in your development. These hormones are pretty powerful. They can regulate your menstrual cycle, aid in muscle development, and repair your body's tissues. You want to grow stronger, right?

I don't want you to worry. There are many ways you can take control of your sleep schedule and rest easy through the night.

It's easier said than done, but I'm going to spell it out for you.

Getting Better Sleep

That was a lot of scary stuff. Don't worry. You have the ability to change your sleep habits and avoid the negative physical and mental effects of poor sleep. We can't necessarily fight our internal clock, but luckily, there are many ways to manage the natural changes happening in our bodies. Let's explore some ways we can cope with these changes. You have the power to use sleep to your benefit. You've got this girl.

How Much Sleep Do You Really Need?

Regardless of what Reddit or TikTok is telling you, you need between eight and ten hours of sleep a night to reap all the amazing benefits of a good night's rest (Gavin, 2019).

You might even think you're getting enough sleep already. Maybe you don't feel the grog and mental fog your friends describe. Maybe you don't even need coffee in the morning. Eight hours is a conservative estimate. If you feel cranky in the morning or have trouble staying awake during your classes, you might need more than eight hours to fully benefit from your sleep.

In fact, studies show that women require about twenty more minutes of sleep nightly than their lame counterparts do (Worley, 2016). Women love to multi-task, we push ourselves. We're flexible. On average, women use more of their brain power daily than men (it's just facts).

You've worked hard to develop your thinking skills. You revel in A's on math tests and you want to have the fastest mile time.

Your brain powers your ability to do what you have to do.

So treat your brain. It does a lot for you.

Developing Healthier Sleep Habits and Staying Awake

It's possible, even though you're a busy gal.

It begins with you.

Begin by setting a regular morning and bedtime routine. If you need to leave home at 7 AM to arrive at school on time, consider what time you need to wake up to be ready. If you have to brush your teeth, pick out clothes, make a decent breakfast, and apply some mascara, you probably need to wake up close to 6 AM.

Do this daily. It's a routine. It's tempting to sleep until noon on the weekends to recuperate that extra rest, but this habit is a temporary fix. You must develop the habit of waking up at the same time every day to reap the benefits of a healthy sleep schedule.

Count back from there. If you know you need 8.5 hours of sleep nightly, you have to go to bed around 9:30 PM to get that rest.

It takes your body time to get used to a sleep schedule. After you figure out the times that work for you, stick to them. It's hard at first; you might find yourself tossing back and forth at 9:30 the first few nights. But it will get easier. Hold yourself accountable.

Try napping responsively. Naps get a bad rep, and for the most part, they're hindering your sleep schedule. You might be an avid napper or you may hate them all together, but like them or not, taking excessive naps can impair your ability to fall asleep at the time you've decided. Nap more responsibly and use them to your advantage. Napping for more than twenty minutes can impair your sleep schedule, so stick to that timeframe.

Use naps to treat yourself. If you've had a particularly hard practice, treat yourself with a little catnap. But try to stick to the twenty-minute rule. Don't nap every day, use them as a reward.

Before going to bed, take an hour or so to unplug and relax. If you have to be in bed by 9:30, plug in your phone and stop scrolling by 8 PM at the latest. Think about the impact of screen time on your beauty sleep. You deserve rest, so take the last hour of the day to reflect and relax in a way that works for you.

If you like meditation or journaling, use that extra hour to do some exercises. If you like knitting or reading, do that. Use this time to benefit you. It's not meant to be a punishment. I'm not saying that extra screen time isn't fun or exciting. But you have to prioritize yourself and your body. Treat it as a little well-deserved break.

Try eating a healthy snack to cope with the fatigue. Don't reach for a candy or chocolate bar (unless it's your period, of course). Try eating a healthy fruit or vegetable snack to keep your brain active. Consuming nutrients throughout the day is important to regulate your sleep patterns. Staying awake isn't easy, but with a little self-help, it's possible.

Before you reach for the coffeemaker, try some deep breathing exercises. It sounds counterintuitive, but breathing and meditation are great ways to regulate your sleep-wake cycle. Again, it's science.

Doing deep breathing exercises helps your body oxygenate your blood (Peri, 2009). Your heart rate slows, and so does your breathing. Slowing down your heart rate and giving your blood cell enough oxygen can allow you to relax a bit and provides you with the energy boost you need to get through the day.

Try some of these tips to get better sleep. After reading, you should be able to recognize the importance of sleep and how it affects your body. Use sleep to your advantage and take control of your daily life.

It's easier said than done, but you are in control of your health.

Period Pennings

End the chapter by answering some of these questions and filling in the blanks. Use your answers to understand why you might be feeling anxious about adopting better habits. Reflect on what you've learned and apply it to your life.

- I get _____ hours of sleep right now. To feel more energized and to reach my goals, I need to get _____ hours of sleep instead.
- _____, _____, and _____ have been keeping me up lately. I feel _____ about it.
- I know that adopting a healthier sleep routine will benefit me in _____ way.
- Starting now, I can try doing _____to better my sleep habits.

Chapter 3: Let's Talk Fashion & Nutrition

Ahh, fashion. You may love it, follow it, *breathe* it, or you may reject it altogether. No matter your personal style, it's important to dress in a way that makes you feel confident and happy.

Being true to your style is key to cultivating confidence. But remember — your style may absolutely change as you enter this new and exciting phase in your life. At some point, you'll stop wearing training bras and wear different ones (maybe ones with padding or an underwire!). Over time, you may feel more confident in heels than you would in light-up sneakers. Maybe you'll always love sneakers!

Whatever the case may be, your personal style will change over time as you grow and develop. It's nothing to be afraid of. Being stylish and confident doesn't have to mean a specific thing: style is about being true to yourself.

Nevertheless, as your body changes, your style will likely change. As your breast and hips develop, you'll find new clothes and undergarments to flatter your changing body.

Even more, the way you feed and take care of your body will likely change as well. Your tastes may change after you experience your first period and your body will grow

31

dramatically. Remember, good nutrition and eating habits never go out of style.

Let's begin by exploring the way style has evolved over the past century, and what this means for what you wear today.

Style Through The Ages

You probably know a little about popular styles in the past. When you think of the 1920s, do you think of the flapper girl with bobbed hair and tassel dresses? When you think of the 1980s, do you think about leg warmers, Madonna, and bright colors?

Think about popular styles from the past. In this section, we'll discuss not only the styles and clothing popular during the last century, but we'll discuss how these fads reflected the styles of teenage girls.

In the Roaring 20s

Clara Bow with her bobbed hair and dark lipstick was an icon of the twenties. Young girls flocked to the nearest hairdresser to achieve the popular flapper hairstyle and wore dark makeup to exaggerate their angular features.

This decade was characterized by a break from Victorian fashion, which was rigid and laced up with corsets. Fashion in the roaring twenties was meant to be freeing and almost androgynous in nature. Clothing was darker and more dramatic, with dropped waistlines and exposed ankles (shocking!).

During this decade, young girls (just your age) wanted to emulate the sophisticated adult style they saw on the silver screen. They looked up to older women and sought to dress just like them. Many young girls would roll up their stockings and dare to wear dresses with shorter hemlines.

Think about your style today. Do you try to dress older than your age? It's okay to be honest, many girls do! Your mother or older sisters might influence your style. You might try out different makeup techniques or wear outfits with lower necklines.

I remember watching my mother apply her lipstick before a date night with family friends. I admired the detail and care she took to look her best. She loves bright prints and pastel colors, so growing up, I did the same!

Consider the people who influence your personal style and reflect on how their fashion sense has affected your own.

The 1930s and "Sub-Deb" Style

The Great Depression of the late 1920s and 1930s inspired a great deal of change in the fashion industry. In a time of widespread unemployment and poverty, many young girls admired high society and unattainable wealth.

The upper class and their style heavily influenced clothing in the 1930s. The style was called "sub-deb," short for "sub debutante." If you're unfamiliar with the word, never fear! The term sub-deb referred to young girls in high society who were preparing for their formal debut (Glamour, 2020).

Women dressed older than their age, but their dresses maintained traditionally youthful touches, like fringed collars and bows. Silhouettes were longer and sleeker than those popular in the decade before; most dresses fell below the knee.

As noted, upper-class fashion heavily influenced the style in this decade. Think about your style today. Are you influenced by wealthy idols like Kylie Jenner or Addison Rae? On some level, probably.

The 1940s and Teenage Fashion

The New York Times coined the term "teenage" in 1945 and referred to those between the ages of thirteen and nineteen. WWII heavily influenced styles, and rations for clothing caused certain materials to become quite limited. Sweater sets that could be made at home became more popular and women adopted new, easily accessible styles.

Teenagers opted to wear bobby socks, ankle-length socks, saddle shoes, or early forms of sneakers. These allowed them to move more freely and casually and to be more active in activities. In fact, teenage girls who adopted this style were called "bobby soxers" because of their interest in popular music (Glamour, 2020).

Again, think about how these influences might affect your own style. Do you dress differently when performing certain activities? Do you try to remain comfortable? Probably. This decade represents the importance of using the clothes and resources available to your advantage.

Return to the Norm: Style in the 50s

The 1950s were a time of joy and change. Women returned to some of the style influences popular in the 1930s and skirts became fuller as materials became readily available following the Second World War.

Women adopted a more feminine style as society entered a period of drastic progress and growth. Teenagers enjoyed bright floral prints with high necklines because of an increased focus on modesty. The style became more rigid as people worked laboriously to return to the pre-war lifestyle.

The Swingin' Sixties and 1970s Counterculture

The 1960s were a time of drastic social change. Women and minority rights were at the forefront of society and influenced fashion accordingly. The term "youthquake," coined by the at-the-time Editor and Chief of Vogue, Diana Vreeland, referred to the mass influence of teen interests on fashion.

Music became bouncier, skirts were shorter, and necklines were more daring. The style became more rebellious and free. The 1960s saw the introduction of miniskirts, which are still quite popular today.

The media was a huge influence on fashion. Stars like Marilyn Monroe and Twiggy embraced their feminine power, causing younger women to do the same.

In the 1970s, style grew much more casual. Pants became a staple to a teenager's wardrobe, and denim grew in popularity. Fashion grew slightly more gender neutral, as both men and women opted for easily accessible clothing styles.

In these decades, fashion represented a break from the norm as women gained more rights and freedoms.

I ask you once again to reflect on what influences your own style. Many young women spend their teen years breaking from the norm and embracing popular and sometimes daring new styles. Does this apply to you?

The 80s and 90s: Introduction to the "Teen Dream"

The 1980s were colorful, casual, and fun. Floral prints and bright colors soared in popularity, as did colorful makeup. Teenagers embraced their femininity and were inspired by popular movies, including *The Breakfast Club* and *Pretty In Pink*. Molly Ringwald and Madonna became fashion icons, inspiring women to dress in a feminine and fun manner.

Pop culture was a huge influence on style at the time. Music, movies, and TV shows were at the center of teenage life. The accessibility of television shows and listening devices caused widespread interest in popular culture and movies.

The term "teen dream" was coined in the 1990s. Movies like *Clueless* and the TV show *Friends* illustrated a sort of cookie-cutter style and fashion. Movies illustrated the perceived importance of being popular, pretty, and wealthy. Teenagers experienced pressure to look a certain way, and this contributed to the rise of diet culture.

Women were pressured to show off their bodies. Skirts got shorter, shirts grew smaller, and clothes grew tighter as women learned to embrace their femininity.

This pressure wasn't without its faults. The 1990s introduced the dangerous idea that teens not only had to dress a certain way, but had to be a certain size to fit into the norm. The rates of certain eating disorders soared as women tried to become more cookie cutter.

Heading into the 2000s

Most of you were born somewhere in the 2000s, and might remember the styles popular during that time. The 2000s saw a rise in the term "tween," referring to girls between the ages of ten and thirteen. Tweens were characterized by their fun, sparkly, funky style. They embraced their age and body type through lip gloss, hair barrettes, and neon shorts. Accessories were king and grew in popularity.

Think about the way you accessorize your own wardrobe. Do you like headbands, colorful hair ties, or bracelets?

2010s: The VSCO Era

You probably remember this style and fashion trend quite well. Maybe you yourself were a "VSCO girl." The rise in social media platforms influenced the 2010s and early 2020s style, including Instagram, Twitter, Tumblr, and VSCO. The influencers they saw inspired teens online, and tried to be as cookie-cutter as possible, much like teens in the 90s.

VSCO style rose in popularity. This trend was characterized by cool, comfy clothes, including scrunchies, denim shorts, big t-shirts, Birkenstock sandals, and large Hydroflask water bottles. The VSCO girl cared about popular trends in an uncaring way. They seemed to reject notions of high-class style, while still holding onto certain expensive accessories.

The emphasis on comfort flowed into the 2020s with ease. The COVID-19 pandemic saw an increase in the popularity of sweatsuit sets, comfy shorts, and neutral colors. TikTok stars like Addison Rae and Charli D'Amelio were responsible for the influx of dyed hair trends and a "don't care" attitude.

So How Does Style Affect Teens?

Just like teens over the last century, trends and cultural changes probably influenced your style. I asked you to consider some ways you're influenced by certain styles and how these affect your own sense of self.

So what really affects your sense of style? Let's talk.

Peer Pressure

In my experience, peer pressure is the most important factor and influence on a teen's individual style. You might not recognize it, but it's likely peer pressure affects your life in many different, and sometimes negative, ways.

Think about this: Your best friend comes to school wearing a matching light blue Lululemon athletic set (if it's within your school's dress code, of course). She gets compliments from boys, other acquaintances, and maybe even a teacher or two. You feel a tinge of envy every time she gets noticed, and you want to be noticed too!

So you beg your mother for the same matching set. If Lululemon is out of your budget, you try Marshalls or TJMaxx to find one just like hers. Your mother or guardian *finally* caves and buys you the set. You feel happy, comfortable, and welcome. You go to school and get the same compliments (maybe even one from your crush!) and you feel a sense of joy and satisfaction.

You experienced peer pressure. Think about your friend group. You all likely have a similar style, right?

Many young teens "presume that if they dress in an inappropriate manner, their peers would not want to interact or socialize with them" (McQuenzie, 2020). It's human. We want to replicate the styles we see around us and ward off what we perceive to be "bad attention."

I'm not asking you to suddenly abandon your style simply because you're inspired by those around you; I'm asking you to think about the ways you may feel pressured to dress a certain way. Reflect on why you love shopping at Shein or Lulu's.

Body Image and Media

It's likely that, in some way, your style is influenced by how you see your body. Again, it's okay to know this, but you have to be conscious of it.

Many teens are embarrassed by their growing breasts or hips, especially if they're early bloomers. If you feel you fall into this category, you might feel pressured to wear baggy tops or large sweatshirts to mask your developing body.

We're influenced by what we see on social media. Think about the models on the cover of magazines. Whether or not you know it, you're influenced by the Hadid sisters or Kendall Jenner. We want to be what we see.

We can't compare ourselves to others. Everyone has their own unique body shape and type. We all come from different ethnic and cultural backgrounds that influence the way we look, and that's something to celebrate.

We don't really know what those models did to look the way they do, and they certainly have Photoshop on their side.

We can't compare ourselves to the norm. We have to compare ourselves to ourselves.

Celebrity Culture

Teens and young women have looked up to celebrities as style icons since the rise in mass media. Even in the 1920s, young girls tried to emulate the style and look of actress Clara Bow. This hasn't changed in recent years.

Think about the celebrities you admire. I'm a fan of Jennifer Lawrence's casual style myself. We're surrounded by reality TV, photos, and Instagram posts from celebrities, and these images affect the way we dress and present ourselves. We have to be conscious of this admiration.

Celebrities have access to stylists, trainers, designers, plastic surgeons, and resources we simply don't have access to. It's okay to feel a little discouraged when you see a famous model sporting a designer bag or high cheekbones. We have to remember that we can only make the most of what we have. And I guarantee you, with a little creativity, you can be your own style icon.

Brands and Designers

Gucci, Prada, Louis Vuitton, Armani; who do you think of when you think of designers? Designer brands influence our style in ways we might not even consider. Every season, designers display their collections, and the colors and styles they present trickle down to the brands you purchase all the time.

Designer clothing or accessories are a status symbol. The Hermes Birkin displays wealth and luxury. Cartier love bracelets illustrate sophistication. You might be drawn to clothing with brand labels. Most people are because they illustrate a sense of perceived wealth.

We want to be "cool" and we want to seem sophisticated. No matter your sense of style, you likely look up to those who sport designer bags and sunglasses. And that's okay.

Be conscious of the ways media, brands, peer pressure, and body image affect your personal style. Reflect on what you think style means to you.

The Negative Effects of the Fashion Industry

There are many negative effects of societal pressure to dress a certain way or appear a certain way. During an age of mass media exposure, it's difficult to filter what positively or negatively affects the way we view ourselves. To overcome these negative influences, we have to first be conscious of them.

Recent studies show that those participating in the fashion industry are 25% more likely to experience mental illnesses, including depression, anxiety, or anorexia nervosa (Griffin, 2020). Models often feel extreme pressure from designers and agencies to appear tall, thin, and blemish-free. That kind of pressure can take a serious toll on one's mental health.

It doesn't stop there. Those who obsess over popular trends and looks can experience a similar feeling. If you don't look like the women you're told are traditionally beautiful, it's hard to feel attractive. Peer pressure is a powerful thing. Comparing yourself to your friends who may fit traditional beauty standards is dangerous.

Traditional beauty standards are just that; traditional. Traditions can be changed or broken over time. For a while, it was the tradition that women forgo wearing pants. You probably wear pants most of the time!

Fashion changes; it changes all the time. Think about the

styles that were popular fifteen years ago. You probably wouldn't be caught wearing low-rise jeans or slouchy bedazzled hats.

The transient nature of the fashion industry can be negative, too. The fashion industry furthers what's known as consumerism, or the preoccupation with wanting more. Again, it's human nature to want what we don't have. Because fashion and popular styles change rapidly, we feel a certain pressure to buy the new, hottest thing.

It isn't good for your wallet, and it's even worse for your mental health.

Think about the first outfit you bought or found for yourself. It was probably a few years ago. You spent a lot of time (or money) finding the outfit and making it "work." Did wearing that outfit make you feel good? Probably; at least for a little while. Did it give you long-term satisfaction? Probably not.

Fashion has likely changed since then. The new outfit you'd saved for doesn't fit the style norm today. Now, you feel pressured to buy a new pair of mom jeans or a certain two-piece track set. It's a cycle of neverending pressure that's hard to swallow.

So how do you overcome this pressure? It's difficult but doable. Cultivating classic clothing pieces that make you feel good is a good place to start. Develop a style that makes you feel good about yourself. This style may change over time, and that's alright! Instead of focusing on what's popular, focus on what makes you happy.

Style and Self-Expression

Enough with the heavy. Style is a powerful way to illustrate your own self-expression. As a teen, your style might go through phases. While I was becoming an adult, I went through a phase where I sported black clothing and chain bracelets. After that, I loved high heels and fitted skinny jeans. As I entered my late teens and early twenties, I valued comfort and sorority labels.

Style is a means of expressing your own creativity. You might not be familiar with the show *F.R.I.E.N.D.S.*, so I'll explain. In the show, the female lead Rachel goes through a style evolution that turns into an exciting career opportunity. She loves sleek outfits and form-fitting tops. At the beginning of the sitcom, she's a waitress at a coffee establishment, but her style leads her to an opportunity to be a Fashion Buyer and Personal Shopper at Bloomingdale's. Eventually, she was offered an executive position at Ralph Lauren and Louis Vuitton.

We take a lot of time trying new styles and brands. It's fun! You might express yourself through haircuts, accessories, new vibes, and certain colors. It's great to express yourself through your clothing, and it's to be encouraged.

What you wear and how you present yourself is a piece of who you are. Don't be afraid to be honest!

The Ins and Outs of Bras

For me, breast development was the most exciting part of puberty. I wanted to look like my mother and the models I saw in magazines. I wanted larger breasts that made me feel like a woman. It's meant to be exciting! Breast development is one of the most important and visible parts of puberty. It's a step your body is taking to become a strong adult!

Breasts begin developing between ages eight and thirteen, but it varies for everyone! You can't make your breasts grow faster, even if you want to. You might feel anxious or discouraged when you look at your friends. Their bodies are on a different clock than yours! It's okay to be a late bloomer or an early developer. Every body is different.

Also remember, breasts don't grow overnight. You won't suddenly wake up with a C cup. That's okay. Breast development takes time, and it may look different for everyone. In some teens, one breast might be slightly larger than the other. Other people have breasts that are more pointy and others' breasts are more round. That's fine.

Your body is unique to you.

Breast development is based on a variety of factors, including genetics and diet. If your mother or older sister began growing breasts at age eleven, it's likely you will too. But don't fear. It's also quite common for your breasts to look entirely different from your mother's (Gavin, 2018). My mother has particularly large breasts, as do my sister and grandmother. I have smaller and more rounded breasts. It's okay to feel a certain amount of anxiety about the way they look. But don't worry. Your body is beautiful no matter what.

This brings us to bras. You might feel apprehensive or nervous about them, but no matter how you feel, bras are a great tool to make you feel better about your clothes.

Types of Bras

Lucky for us, there are many different types of bras to fit your activity level, clothing style, and body type. Let's explore the different bras and what they do for you!

Training Bras

Training bras serve as your starter bra. They're your introduction to wearing a bra. The point of a training bra isn't necessary to achieve a certain look or support level; the point is to teach you how to wear a bra.

A training bra looks similar to a sports bra, but doesn't provide the same level of support. They're often made of thin, cotton material that protects your growing nipples from chafing against your clothing. They can have thin or thick adjustable straps and may have a clasp or an elastic to hold the bra in place.

So when are you ready for a training bra? That's up to you! Before purchasing a training bra, ask yourself these questions.

- Have you started developing breast buds?
- Do you feel self-conscious when you wear a thin t-shirt?
- Do you engage in activities that might call for a little more support?

If you've answered yes to even one of these questions, it might be time to consider buying a training bra.

After you get used to wearing a bra, there are many other options available to you based on the look you desire and your body type. Let's dive in!

Padded Bras

When you think about bras, you likely think of padded bras. These are among the most common types and come in a variety of styles and shapes.

Padded bras are just that: Bras with padding. They contain a small insert or built-in cup that adds volume to your breasts. Padded bras can come with an underwire or without, and you can choose a style that's comfortable for you.

Padded bras work for women with any breast size or shape. You can wear them every day and with most types of clothing.

Push-Up Bras

Push-up bras are a type of padded bra with a boost. They often contain an underwire or extra support. Most push-up bras have extra padding to gently press your breast together for a more dramatic appearance. There are different levels of push-up bras, and they're meant to make your breasts appear larger.

The majority of women who choose padded bras tend to have smaller breasts and they're meant to be worn with lower-cut tops or dresses.

This is a bit of a disclaimer. You don't need to run to your nearest Victoria's Secret and splurge on a Bombshell bra.

Don't feel pressured to wear a push-up bra too soon; there's no rush. Push-up bras are meant for special occasions, and oftentimes you might want to wait a bit before purchasing one. Embrace your body before making any changes.

Convertible Bras

Convertible bras may or may not contain padding, but are meant to provide flexibility. The straps on convertible bras can be altered. The straps can be changed to cross in the back, form a halter neckline, or be worn in the traditional way. This allows you more flexibility when choosing new clothing.

Convertible bras can come with a bit of a learning curve. I remember getting ready for prom and struggling with the little clasps. Practice a few times before wearing a convertible bra.

Convertible bras come in a variety of colors, types, and styles, meaning everyone, no matter your cup size, can wear a convertible bra.

Bralette

Bralettes are a mix between a sports bra and a traditional bra. They're often more decorative, and many appear lacy. Bralettes are not meant for support and shouldn't be worn while engaging in physical activity.

Bralettes are primarily meant for women with smaller breasts, but everyone can wear a bralette! There are many different sizes and types, so feel free to find a style that works for you!

Sports Bras

Sports bras are meant for just that — sports! Sports bras are often quite comfortable and versatile and exist in many styles.

Some sports bras offer padding for additional support, which may help if you have larger breasts. Other sports bras offer lower levels of support and are meant for low-impact activities like walking or yoga.

Sports bras are meant for all women regardless of breast size. They're meant to prevent discomfort during exercise; long-term, sports bras can help protect against sagging.

These are just a few of the many styles and types of bras available. Most girls begin wearing a training bra before graduating to wearing other types of bras. It's important to try different styles to find what works best for you!

Bra Sizes

Finding your bra size is key to finding bras that are comfortable and easily worn. It might seem a little difficult at first, but I'm going to break it down for you.

Remember, your bra size will absolutely change throughout the course of your life. I recommend measuring yourself about once a year until the age of eighteen. If you find your bras don't fit as they normally do, feel free to re-measure any time.

You can also get measured by a professional, which might be helpful at first.

Comfort and fit are important, so prioritize it!

There are two measurements that determine your bra size; your band size and your cup size. The band size refers to where the main band of the bra sits, usually just below your breast. The cup size is the size of the padded or "cupped" part of the bra. You'll measure these two sizes in U.S. inches, and always remember to round up if the measurement falls on an odd number.

Begin by wrapping a measuring tape around the area your bra would sit. Jot down this measurement and round up to an even number if the measurement is odd. Then add four.

So, for example, if you measure your band size and it's 28 inches, your band size measurement would be 32.

Next, put on a bra you currently wear. Your cup measurement can be taken without wearing a bra, but this measurement can be inaccurate at times (we'll get to that later). If you're wearing a bra, make sure it allows space for your breast to breathe. Don't wear a sports bra or anything tight when taking this measurement.

Measure at nipple level and round to the nearest whole number. This number can be odd or even. Jot down the number you get.

Now, subtract your cup size from your band size. Then compare it to the chart I've created below to figure out your true cup size.

So, for example, if you measure your band size and it's 26 inches, add four. Your correct band size is 30. Measure your cup size. Perhaps your cup size is 33 inches. Subtract 33 by 30. Your correct bra size is 30C.

It's okay to get a little confused. If you find the chart difficult, there are many online bra size calculators you can use.

Keep in mind that bra size is variable. It's a little confusing, I'll admit. Think about it this way: A 32B and a 36B are completely different sizes and have nothing to do with the size of your breasts. Someone with a 34D bra size will have a larger cup size (and breast size) than someone whose size is 28D. It's perfectly normal!

Always remember: Try it on! Every retailer is different. Make sure to try on bras in the store before purchasing them. Size charts are very important, and every bra is different depending on the style and type.

Don't feel discouraged about your bra size. Your body is growing and changing, and it's likely your bra size will too. Don't feel upset if your friend is a 36DDD and your size is 32B. Everyone is different. Owning and wearing the correct bra can make or break a cute outfit.

Bras and growing breasts are an important part of becoming a woman. It's okay to feel a little anxious or uncomfortable at first. That's perfectly normal. Your body is changing, and change is hard. Focus on the positives — you're becoming the strong woman you were meant to be. Embrace your body, no matter the size or shape.

Good Nutrition Never Goes Out of Style

Taking care of your body by feeding it the right nutrients is more important than what you put it in.

Clothing comes and goes; styles always change. But being and feeling healthy simply don't. The effects of eating healthy last a lifetime, and I doubt your new jeans will.

Whether or not you know it, there is a strong and interesting correlation between food and style. Lori Reamer, the author of *Food That Fits*, found in her research that many of the clients seeking nutritional counseling were "highly connected to their external appearance… these women disliked grocery shopping, owned homes with beautiful kitchens but didn't cook, and had a history of food avoidance to help control weight" (Schlamberg, 2012).

She used this example: "When you tell a woman who's

wearing a beautiful cashmere Ralph Lauren sweater that she's feeding herself the equivalent of poor-quality acrylic fabric, you get quite a reaction," the clients in question, "wouldn't consider wearing low-end acrylic, so why would she tolerate eating that way" (Schlamberg, 2012). As I noted before, jeans, even those of good quality, last a few years, while positive nutritional habits last forever.

Clothing, similar to food, is a symbol of "comfort and pleasure" (Schlamberg, 2012). Food staples, like vegetables or colorful fruits, are nutritional staples, just like a nice black dress or a leather bag. Additionally, just like style, food makes you feel good!

Think about it this way: when you eat a balanced diet, one filled with colorful foods and whole grains, you feel just as good as if you were wearing your best outfit.

The Nutrient Breakdown

You can't follow a healthy diet if you don't understand the requirements, right? Nutritional guidelines aren't a one-size fits all blouse; they're unique to each person. However, a basic understanding of the nutrients and quantities you should consume is a powerful way to begin your healthy diet (and style) journey.

Use the following chart as a guide to understanding your unique nutrient requirements.

Those marked with * may be subject to change based on National Guidelines.

Calorie guidelines are subject to change based on your activity level. Those participating in high-intensity activities (such as gymnastics, track, and field, volleyball, etc.) may require more calories than those who live a less active lifestyle.

Fat is a bit more tricky. I'll explain. Realistically, you need about 8-10 teaspoons of fat daily to maintain your fat guidelines. Believe me, it's less than you'd think. Fat used when cooking adds up over time. Consider making your meals at home to monitor how much fat is really being used. Fats can also come from plant sources, like olive oil or safflower oil. These are called unsaturated fats, as they're liquid at room temperature. Saturated fats, like butter or margarine, should be limited.

Carbohydrates are absolutely essential to your diet. While these guidelines vary from person to person, shooting for about 15 servings of carbohydrates is a good place to start. So what does one serving look like? A single serving of carbohydrates looks like one medium apple or one slice of bread. It's easier than you'd think to hit your carbohydrate goals.

Proteins, just like carbohydrates, are quite important. Again, protein recommendations vary from person to person, but shooting for about 5 ounces of protein daily is a good place to start. A chicken breast, a small handful of nuts, or low-fat dairy products are all good protein sources to help you meet your protein goals.

You should aim for two cups of fruit daily and 2.5 cups of vegetables. Make sure your fruits and veggies are colorful. The coloring in fruits and veggies comes from antioxidants and nutrients necessary for long-term health. It's important to note that both fruits and vegetables are important. You can't substitute a fruit serving for a vegetable serving.

Try to aim for three servings of low-fat dairy per day. A cup of low-fat milk or one ounce of cheese is a good place to start to help you reach your dairy and calcium goals.

Fortified foods or drinks, like fortified orange juice or milk, are good sources of vitamin D. Getting outside will also aid in your body's ability to produce its own vitamin D. Foods like salmon and tuna are also good sources of vitamin D.

Sodium should be kept at a minimum. In the United States, it's unlikely you're lacking in sodium. Consume foods that are flavorful and nutritious. It's likely you're already meeting (or exceeding) your sodium intake goals.

As I said, none of these are cut-and-dry. There is no one-size-fits-all black dress when it comes to nutrition. Mix and match.

Begin by making your plates as colorful as possible and limiting foods like sugary beverages. Try making meals at home to help yourself practice.

I'm not saying you should download a calorie and macro tracking app. In fact, apps like MyFitnessPal perpetuate dangerous ideas about what a person "should" and "shouldn't" eat. Use the information provided as a guide to help you understand the role nutrition plays in your health.

It's okay to falter, and it's okay to treat yourself. Remember, everything exists in moderation. Feed your body. It's yours forever.

Period Pennings

Fill in these blanks to help gauge your understanding of your own style and nutritional health. Remember, this is about you. You don't have to fit a certain "mold" to be healthy and stylish. Style changes all the time. Be your best you.

- I love wearing _____ and _____ because these pieces make me feel confident.
- I feel that _____, _____, and _____ influence my unique style.
- I think my aesthetic is _____ and I find it makes me feel _____ way.
- I love eating _____ because it makes me feel good. I also like eating _____ because I feel it fuels my body.
- My diet might be lacking in _____ or _____. I plan to eat more _____ and perhaps less of _____ to help me meet my nutrient goals.

Chapter 4: You're Beautiful

Every body is beautiful. Read that as many times as you'd like.

Body positivity is a habit and practice, but that doesn't mean it's always easy. In a world full of naysayers and mass media, it can be difficult to accept your body as it is.

You've probably heard of the body positivity movement by now. Stars like Lizzo, Selena Gomez, and Ashley Graham all preach the importance of loving yourself as you are. The body positivity movement challenges the way society views certain body types, promotes widespread acceptance of all bodies, helps people struggling to build their own confidence, and addresses body standards that are unrealistic (Cherry, 2020). It's important, especially during your teens, to develop an acceptance of the body you have.

Unfortunately, body positivity presents a sort of caveat. At its core, the body positivity movement supports the notion that every body is beautiful. And, of course, that's true.

Think about the wording in the phrase, "every body is beautiful." Many scientists and social psychologists believe the body positivity movement emphasizes the notion that a person's worth is directly related to how they look.

It doesn't have to be that way. Body image is comprehensive

and directly tied to one's confidence and sense of self-worth. Body image should be looked at as a collection of who you are, not simply a summary of how you look.

Forming a positive self-image takes time, but it's absolutely possible. Let's explore the ins and outs of loving the body you were born with.

You Aren't Alone

If you feel uncomfortable in your own skin, don't fear. You certainly aren't alone; many women and especially teens, struggle with accepting their bodies. In fact, most adult women, whether or not they admit it, have a difficult relationship with their bodies. I certainly did!

And it starts much younger than you'd think.

Allure Magazine compiled a series of interviews with girls between the ages of six and eighteen who discuss how they feel about their bodies. Each girl shared her personal discomforts with their physical features. Many discussed certain societal pressures that drove or aggravated their relationship with their bodies.

Think about the "thigh gap" trend popular a few years ago. I remember this one vividly, but if you don't, that's okay. In the early 2010s, Tumblr was responsible for perpetuating images of teenage girls with what's called a thigh gap, or a small space between their legs shown when their feet are pressed together. To get a "thigh gap," one had to be extremely thin; many women simply weren't built to have a thigh gap, no matter their weight.

This is just a small example of a more widespread social issue; many body standards are simply unattainable, regardless of height and weight. It can be discouraging. If your body simply can't or won't fit into a specific body standard, like the thigh gap, you might become anxious or worried.

Over the past century, many body standards have grown and receded in popularity, and they're nearly impossible to keep up with.

In the 1950s, a curvier, Marilyn Monroe bombshell body was popular. Women wanted larger breasts and smaller waists to attain that standard of beauty and went to extreme lengths to get there.

The 1980s are another example; the fitness industry grew rapidly and an athletic, toned, yet still slender body became popular. Fitness and aerobics video sales went through the roof and icons like Jane Fonda perpetuated unhealthy beauty standards regarding personal fitness.

In the 1990s, women wanted to be wafer-thin, like supermodel Kate Moss. This was similarly unattainable for many. Most people aren't built to appear super-skinny, no matter the number on the scale.

In the 2020s, the thigh gap isn't very popular.

Instead of the thigh gap, women aspire to be what's called "slim-thick." Slim thick refers to a body that's thick in the "right" places, primarily the butt and thighs, but that's slender in the waist.

Again, this simply isn't attainable. The slim-thick body standard perpetuates feelings of discouragement and negatively affects women of all sizes. Teens who are naturally thin struggle to feel comfortable because they feel their butt is too small or their thighs are too slender. Women who have larger body types might feel as though their waist or arms are too big.

It's a facade. No matter your size, this standard isn't attainable.

Coping and Fitting Into The Unattainable

Girls as young as ten years old feel a certain pressure to appear thinner or have larger feminine features. In one of the interviews, a ten-year-old girl describes wearing black leggings and tells the interviewer she does so to make herself appear thinner.

I fell into this trap, too. Throughout my early 20s, I wore almost exclusively black for its "slimming" effect. I don't think I looked much slimmer. In fact, I probably looked dressed for a funeral.

Many of the girls interviewed mentioned comparing themselves to their super-skinny friends. Teens want to fit in, but "fitting in" is virtually impossible; especially when there are so many different body types and sizes.

Other girls in the *Allure* interview, ones as young as ten, tell the interviewer they don't look in the mirror to avoid feeling discouraged. This is more common than you'd think; many of my friends growing up would avoid dressing or fitting rooms because of the full-length mirror.

But it's not just about being a certain weight or having certain proportions. Many girls feel self-conscious about their height, or lack thereof. Taller girls may slouch to appear shorter than they are, while shorter teens may stand up straighter and wear shoes that make them look taller.

It's difficult not to compare yourself to others. We notice when those around us are particularly thin; it's hard to ignore. Comparison is the killer of confidence, and to be confident, we have to find things about ourselves to admire or like.

Comparisons are dangerous. They lead to obsessions that can cause negative long-term effects on your life.

You might be familiar with certain eating disorders. Disordered eating can arise when one experiences extreme shame in the body they were born with. I won't go into specifics, but disorders like anorexia nervosa and bulimia nervosa are difficult to treat and even more difficult to live with.

It's likely you know people who struggle with eating disorders, and we'll discuss these in more detail later in this chapter. Many of my friends in college admitted to suffering from eating disorders. They would fast throughout the day, only to binge eat pizza or candy at night. They stressed over the number on the scale, regardless of how they looked in the mirror.

Outside Comments: The "Good" and the "Ugly"

Have you heard of the term "fat shaming"?" It's likely you have. Fat shaming involves making comments or acting in a way that negatively comments on specific body types, ultimately determining them to be "lesser than." If you've experienced fat shaming, it likely didn't feel good.

But it's been around a long time. I was often body-shamed in middle and high school; girls around me would comment on the size of my thighs and call them "disproportionate" to the rest of my body. They weren't. That's just how I was built.

But I took their comments to heart and felt inadequate. If I'm being honest, I still struggle to forget those comments.

And compliments don't really help. If your parents tell you, "That makes you look skinny," or a friend mentions, "Wow, you look hot," you might feel good at the moment. But do you feel good later? Probably not. In fact, a lot of comments pointed at your body might make you feel judged or watched, even if they're positive.

Outside compliments don't really make a difference, at least not until you believe them yourself.

If those around you make uncomfortable comments about your body, shut them out. Leave them be. Make new friends. Those people aren't helping you to accept yourself. They aren't making you better.

I know it's upsetting. It's hard. It's frustrating.

Remember, the problem isn't with your body. The problem lies in the world around it.

What Even Is Body Image?

Body image "refers to how an individual sees their own body and how attractive they feel themselves to be" (Brazier, 2020). Body image doesn't have to do with just size or shape; body image encompasses how you look and includes hair color, eye color, or even the shape of your nose.

Your body image can change over time. Maybe you've found that it's changed over the past few years.

I used to be quite self-conscious about the shape of my nose. I felt it was too big, too pointy, and too long. Over time, I grew confident in the shape of my nose. I didn't feel like changing it. It's unique and interesting. It took practice, but now, I can honestly say I love my nose.

Body image can be positive or negative. Those with a positive body image feel satisfied and comfortable in their bodies. They're able to discern the parts of themselves they like and why and they're able to accept their body as just parts, not all, of their identity.

Those suffering from a negative body image may be overly critical of the way they look. They might feel self-conscious and might try to change their appearance. They might even have a distorted image of themselves, which is when they think they look a certain way that's not quite accurate.

So which one do you feel applies to you? Are you happy and confident in your skin? If so, that's great. It's equally okay to feel negative about certain parts of yourself. It's normal. You're still growing and changing. You can take the steps necessary to improve your body image.

It's about you.

The Aspects of Body Image

Before diving into what affects your body image, it's important to understand the four aspects of body image. Let's break it down.

- **Perceptual body image** is the way you *see* your body. Unfortunately, it's not always an accurate representation of how you look.
- **Affective body image** refers to how you *feel* about your body. Are you happy with the way you feel you look? Are you disgusted or embarrassed?
- **Cognitive body image** is the way you *think* about your body. This aspect can lead to a preoccupation with your body shape.
- **Behavioral body image** refers to the habits you engage in as a result of how you see yourself. If you feel embarrassed about how you look, you might avoid certain social activities or sports.

These four aspects play a distinct role in the way we see

61

ourselves (National Eating Disorders Collaboration, 2021). We'll cover this in more detail later in the chapter. For now, consider how these aspects affect your body image.

How do you view specific features, like your hips or eye color?

Do you feel positively or negatively about your body? This could refer to any of your features, including your size, shape, profile, or hair color.

What do you think about your body? Do you think it's cool and useful? Do you find it cumbersome and useless?

How do you use your body and treat it? Do you isolate yourself when you feel upset about your body?

What Affects Body Image?

Many things. There are a wide variety of factors that can positively or negatively affect the way you see yourself. These factors include the following.

- social media
- peers and parents
- sports and activities
- puberty
- self-esteem

We've discussed the effects of social media on your body image. It's usually not positive. Images of celebrities and models available online are unattainable. Oftentimes, they're not real. Celebrities have photoshop and perfect lighting at their disposal. They look differently online than they do in real life.

When you look in the mirror, you simply can't photoshop what you see. Remember that. Don't beat yourself up if you don't look like Gigi Hadid or the models you admire. They've been exercising and dieting and altering their bodies for years.

Your peers and parents play a large role in your own body image. We discussed the negative effects of peer pressure and "fitting in" in the previous section, but we haven't discussed your parents and their role in your body image.

Sometimes our parents and guardians are encouraging. They make comments that make you feel good about yourself and they model their own behavior. No matter their own appearance, they exercise a positive influence on our body image.

Unfortunately, not all parents are encouraging when it comes to their children's bodies. My own parents fell into this category.

Growing up, I didn't look like my cousins or my siblings. My mother would show me dresses she wore in her early twenties and encouraged me to try them on. Most of the time, they didn't even zip up.

She praised my younger sister for her slim physique and dark, straight hair, but encouraged me to exercise and tone down my blonde frizz.

My grandmother called me "the ugly duckling," and stressed to my mother the difficulties she'll face while raising an incorrigible child like myself.

My father did the same. When I ate a piece of pizza, he'd remind me of the number of carbs in a slice. He bought me workout clothes for birthdays and he offered to help me make a diet plan.

He thought his efforts would encourage me to lose weight. Guess what? They didn't.

If you feel your experience aligns with mine, I apologize.

63

But I learned to encourage myself. It wasn't easy. In fact, it was really freaking hard. I had to pick out the parts of myself I *did* like, and focus on those. We'll get into ways to improve your body image later. For right now, just remember: you deserve to be surrounded by positive, encouraging people.

Believe it or not, certain sports and activities can play a role in your body image. Teens who engage in dance, gymnastics, or theater might feel a certain pressure to lose weight to get certain roles or master certain skills.

Additionally, teens who play soccer or softball may idolize a more muscular body type. Your ability to perform well doesn't equate to the way your body looks. Venus and Serena Williams aren't slender athletes, but they beat their competition nearly every time.

Puberty & Perception

Newsflash: Puberty plays an important role in how you view yourself. Before puberty, our bodies are still child-like. Our breasts haven't developed, our shoulders are slender, and we don't have obvious waists.

You've probably noticed the way your body's changed since or during puberty. Your hips widen, your bottom half grows, and your breasts get larger. It's all normal. Your body is preparing for adulthood.

Puberty weight gain is perfectly normal. Most women, if not all, gain a considerable amount of weight during their early and mid-teens. It's okay. Don't panic.

Remember, your body is getting ready for womanhood. You wouldn't want to look like a child forever, right?

Self-esteem is a bit more complicated. Self-esteem is influenced by many factors, but we're talking about its role in your body image. If you feel good about yourself and your physical features, you likely have a more positive view of your body. If you feel lacking in intelligence or certain sports, it's likely that you have a negative body image.

Many teens begin to compare their bodies to those of their peers around this time. I remember watching other girls whose bodies fit perfectly into the XS leotards in dance class. I watched my friends' bodies grow faster than mine and I felt a pang of jealousy in the locker room.

It's difficult, but worth it. Abandon the comparisons.

Your perception of your body is yours. Luckily, you have the power to change it.

Reclaim Your Uniqueness

Our bodies are diverse. They come in different shapes, colors, and sizes. Your genetics and family background play a large role in the way your body looks. We discussed breasts in the previous chapter, but think about your body as a whole. If your mother and sisters have wide hips and broad shoulders, you probably will as well.

That's okay. In fact, it's to be celebrated! We come from a variety of backgrounds, and these backgrounds affect the way we look today. Our ancestors, no matter where they were from, developed certain body shapes and sizes to cope with their environment. It's pretty cool. Your culture and ethnic background are important, so celebrate the body it gave you.

Some parts of our bodies are simply out of our control. You might feel dissatisfied with your eye color or breast size. Unfortunately, there's not much we can do about that.

There are parts of our bodies that are within our control. If you feel you lack muscle definition, you can change that by heading to the gym or exercising at home!

There are things we can control and things we simply cannot. Learn to accept and love the parts of your body that you cannot change, and learn your power to change the parts you can.

Have compassion for yourself. Treat your body as you'd like a friend to treat theirs. Would you want your best friend to obsess about their weight and body shape? Would you want them to feel inadequate? Nope.

So give yourself the same love.

Focus on the whole, not the parts. There are always going to be parts of your body you don't like. Focus on the parts you do like, and use them as a means to improve your body image.

You deserve to feel good about the skin you're in.

Negative Body Image and Its Dangers

Negative body image is just that: negative.

Negative body image relates to the four aspects I discussed in the last sections, but can also involve a heightened understanding or awareness of how your body moves and a misinterpretation of what your body looks like or "should" look like (Stanborough, 2020).

Think back to the *Allure* interview we began with. Negative body image is quite common and difficult to overcome. It begins earlier than you'd think. In fact, studies show that 40-50% of girls in the first and second grades don't like certain parts or areas of their body (Stanborough, 2020).

We've discussed some factors that affect one's body image, including peer and parental pressure, social media, sports and activities, and puberty. Unfortunately, these are the same causes of negative body image.

Sometimes, more than one of these affects our body image, and we fall into a dangerous trap of low self-esteem and poor self-image. Maybe your parents often comment on your weight or your friends mention your frizzy hair. You don't deserve these comments, but it's hard to ignore them.

This is when things get a little more serious.

Eating Disorders

Eating disorders come in a wide variety of forms and look different from person to person. Those suffering from an eating disorder find themselves in a negative and potentially dangerous loop of self-doubt, frustration, and shame. Poor body image isn't the only thing that determines the development of an eating disorder, but it certainly doesn't help. Many people suffering from an eating disorder note they had a negative self-image, which only aggravated the issue. Let's explore a few of the most common eating disorders young women suffer from today.

Anorexia Nervosa

Anorexia nervosa, otherwise known as anorexia, is one of the most well-known eating disorders. It can be very dangerous and may cause negative lifelong physical effects.

Anorexia is characterized by an obsession with weight loss. Those with anorexia take extreme and dangerous measures to lose weight (often weight they don't need to lose) and may restrict calories to a minimum.

Keep in mind that anorexia looks different for everyone suffering from the disorder. Just because someone doesn't look particularly thin doesn't mean they don't suffer from anorexia.

Bulimia Nervosa

Bulimia nervosa, otherwise known as bulimia, is characterized by a cycle of binging and purging. One suffering from bulimia may overeat and feel too full, only to purge the food they ate just after.

Purging can look different from person to person. Some people suffering from bulimia may throw up, while others resort to dangerous levels of physical activity to burn calories.

Bulimia is just as dangerous as anorexia. The sufferer may experience long-term malnutrition or other health conditions as a result of the disorder.

Binge Eating Disorder

Often left out of the conversation on eating disorders is the Binge Eating Disorder, but it is just as painful as the two I discussed earlier.

Someone suffering from a binge eating disorder will often eat large amounts of food in a singular sitting or throughout the day. They often have trouble feeling "full" or satisfied.

These episodes are followed by severe feelings of depression, anxiety, and disgust. Binge eating disorders don't involve purging like bulimia or restriction like anorexia. Keep in mind that they're just as harmful.

I don't want to scare you. It's important to educate yourself about eating disorders to fully understand the value of a positive self-image. Not only that, but you should be able to recognize some signs of anorexia or other eating disorders so that you may seek help.

If you feel you suffer from an eating disorder, please contact the National Eating Disorder Association text or call line: (800) 931-2237.

Negative Self-Image For Those With Special Needs

Those with disabilities or special needs, whether they are psychological or physical, often suffer from negative self-image to a higher degree than their non-disabled counterparts do. Remember, disabilities can be visible or invisible. It's important to note that disabilities affect the sufferer in a wide variety of ways.

Think about social media. Unfortunately, it's quite rare to see people with visible disabilities on the cover of magazines or newspapers. Society's attitudes towards those with disabilities are changing, but not quickly enough.

People suffering from disabilities may experience more discrimination or shameful comments about their bodies than their able-bodied peers. It's not okay. We must be mindful of our words and treat everyone's experiences with the respect they're due.

If you suffer from a disability, know that you are never "less than," and you deserve to feel beautiful in the body you were given.

How Do I Know If I Have A Negative Self-Image?

It's sometimes difficult to tell. You might have a negative self-image and not know it. You might even think it's normal.

If you feel you might suffer from a negative self-image, ask yourself these questions provided by Rebecca Stanborough through *Healthline*.

- Do your feelings about your body interfere with your relationships, school, work, or activities?
- Do you take measures to avoid seeing your body?
- Do you compulsively check and recheck your body? This can involve measuring or weighing yourself or constant examination in the mirror.
- Do you feel the need to apply heavy makeup when you go out in public?
- Do you use baggy clothing to hide your body?
- Do you use unkind language to describe your body?

If you've answered yes to one or more of the questions I posed, you may suffer from a negative self-image. Reflect on why you may feel that way and more importantly, pay attention to the next section, where we'll cover how you can feel more beautiful in your body.

How To Build a Positive Self-Image

You know the dangers of a negative self-image, and maybe you identified your own struggle with a negative self-image. It's okay. You're not alone. We're going to talk it out.

Building a positive self-image is a skill anyone can benefit from. Even if you already feel comfy in your own skin, there is always room for improvement.

Try out some of these tips to build or improve your own self-image. You're enough.

Eat For Fuel, Not For Looks

Think about what you learned about nutrition in Chapter Three. If you've forgotten, go back and take a look. It's possible to pay attention to what and how you eat without falling into dangerous habits.

Think of food as fuel for your body. It's like a car. If you give your diesel truck unleaded gas, it will not run properly and might break down. Your body is the same way. Food allows us to accomplish what we need to do. It fuels our brains and our bodies.

Instead of focusing on how a healthy diet will make you look, focus on how it will make you feel. Consuming healthy and colorful portions regularly is essential for long-term health. Eating in moderation and focusing on eating for feeling is a great way to build your positive self-image.

Keep in mind that a healthy body isn't always a skinny one. Healthy comes in many shapes and sizes. Don't let people determine your health based on how you look. Don't let yourself tell yourself you're unhealthy when your doctor says otherwise.

Give your body what it needs.

Set Reasonable Expectations

Don't hold yourself to the unattainable. No one can be the best at everything. That's simply impossible. It is possible, however, to be the best at one thing but be a little "less best" at another. Maybe you kill it in math class but struggle in English. Maybe you love your hair color but don't love your height.

You can be the best at little things. We can't hold ourselves to model-level standards. Push yourself, but not too hard. You're the best at being you, and that's certainly enough.

Positive Influences

Surround yourself with people who encourage you and make you feel good. If you have a friend who criticizes your haircut, leave them be. They're not helping you feel better about yourself. If your sibling makes fun of you for your weight, set boundaries with them. The people that love and support you are those who will bring you up, not keep you down.

Keep in mind that those who criticize you do it for a reason. The reason isn't you — it's them. Those with negative self-image compare themselves to others to make themselves feel good. They deflect from themselves onto you because *they* don't feel good enough. It's a them problem, not a you problem.

Make friends with people who think positively about themselves. It's infectious! People who encourage themselves will also encourage you.

So surround yourself with positive people who lift you up. Make friends with people you feel good about and who believe in you.

Praise Yourself

Award yourself for everything. Acknowledge the areas of your life you feel good about. This doesn't just mean parts of your body. Your identity is determined by everything you are, including your activities, accomplishments, intellect, and humor. If you find yourself to be particularly smart, acknowledge that. If you think you're great at sports, own it, and if you love the color of your eyes, believe it.

You deserve to feel good enough. Body image doesn't simply refer to your appearance; it refers to who you are as a beautiful human being.

Begin by writing the parts of yourself you like or find noteworthy. It's okay if the list is short at first. Over time, look back at the list. Add to it. Reflect on it. When you feel low, take it out and think about what you've written. Use the list as a tool to build your self-image.

Keep in mind that a positive self-image isn't built overnight. It's a practice and a habit. Be kind to yourself as you do those around you. Practice positive self-image daily. You deserve it.

Period Pennings

That was a heavy chapter. Take a bit of time to reflect on what you've learned. It's probably a lot. Fill in the blanks below and answer the questions to consider how you can change your self-image.

Be positive about your body for yourself. You'll thank yourself later.

- I feel positive about _____, _____, _____, _____, and

_____.

- I want to feel better about _____ and _____ so that I can have a more positive self-image.
- Doing _____ and being around _____ makes me feel good about myself.
- I currently feel _____ about my body. I want to feel _____.
- I deserve to view myself more positively, and I plan to try _____to accomplish that goal.

Chapter 5: Loving Yourself

We know mental health is important. At least, I hope you do. In recent years, mental health and the importance of taking care of it has become a hot-button topic.

And for good reason.

Whether or not you realize it, your mental health affects all areas of your life. When we feel down, those around us pick up on our attitude and demeanor. When we feel anxious or worried, we're more likely to avoid spending time with others or engaging in activities we normally enjoy.

Examine what you know about mental health and think about what it means for you. Your brain is the most important organ in your body. When it's experiencing hardship or mental illness, it can affect your physical wellbeing.

Mental Health and Teens

Have you ever told an adult or older sibling you feel anxious or depressed, only to have them tell you, "That's nothing. Wait until you're my age."

They're wrong.

Contrary to what adults might tell you, mental health can

definitely affect you throughout your teens, and usually well into adulthood. In fact, according to a study published in the *Journal of Abnormal Psychology* in 2019, 50% of lifelong mental illnesses and disorders show symptoms before the age of 17 (*Teen mental health: facts & statistics,* 2019).

In fact, this phenomenon may be worsening. The same publication notes that between 2009 and 2017, "cases of major depression among teens ages sixteen and seventeen rose by an overwhelming 69% and reports from people between the ages of seventeen and twenty-five showed feelings of hopelessness increased by 71% in the same timeframe (*Teen mental health: facts & statistics,* 2019).

Additionally, mental health professionals and members of the medical community have referred to the current rising trend in teens requiring mental health treatment as an epidemic. The cause of this jump is unclear. It could be attributed to the rise of social media platforms, which cause teens to compare themselves to their peers. Perhaps it's the result of "hustle" culture.

For a while, it was quite unusual and taboo to discuss mental health openly. The normalization of these candid conversations could be the cause of this increase, too.

Depression seems to disproportionately affect teenage girls. The same study noted that one-in-five girls between the ages of twelve and seventeen had experienced an episode of major depression within the previous year (*Teen mental health: facts & statistics,* 2019).

I don't want you to be scared. It's important to understand the signs of mental illness and how it can affect the person suffering. No one deserves to feel hopeless or alone. Early diagnosis is important to living a happy, healthy life.

Anxiety: The Killer of Confidence

Stress, in small ways, is healthy. It can push you to meet deadlines, reach your goals, and achieve success. However, not all stress is good stress; in fact, when stress becomes overwhelming, it becomes anxiety.

Anxiety isn't just worrying. Anxiety is a harmful and complex disorder that takes different forms. For the purposes of this book, we'll be discussing anxiety as it relates to Generalized Anxiety Disorder (otherwise known as GAD).

As I said, anxiety in small ways is positive. It becomes negative when it's experienced in a disproportionate amount (Pietro, 2015). Teens suffering from anxiety may experience seemingly large reactions to small mistakes and setbacks. When they're a few minutes late to rehearsal, they might experience a strong physical reaction, including shortness of breath, anger or frustration, and nausea.

Anxiety looks different from person to person. Those suffering from anxiety might feel jittery, experience nightmares or restlessness, or general discomfort (Marner, 2021). You may not experience any of these symptoms above.

Those suffering from anxiety often want to appear "normal" (Hurley, 2017). They can be quite good at hiding it, but may also illustrate some of these "hidden" symptoms.

- irritability
- seemingly uncontrollable outbursts
- isolation from friends and family
- changes in eating patterns
- digestive issues
- changes in academic performance (usually dropping grades

and missed assignments)
- dizziness

It's not just worrying; anxiety is serious, and early intervention and treatment are very important. The longer one suffers from anxiety, the more difficult it can be to treat. Think about the symptoms I stated before. If your grades drop because of your anxiety, they're harder to bring back up. You worry about them. You might feel inadequate. If you isolate yourself from friends and family, it's more difficult to rebuild those relationships.

It's like a snowball: it keeps getting larger and more damaging.

Causes of Anxiety

Just like your height and weight, the development of anxiety depends on a variety of factors; including your environment and genetic makeup.

Professionals have varying ideas of the cause of anxiety; sometimes teens develop anxiety with seemingly no cause. Most professionals agree genetics and heredity can trigger that anxiety. It's likely that, if you suffer from anxiety, there are other members of your family that do as well. Additionally, those who develop anxiety might have family members who suffer from other mental health disorders, including Depression, Attention Deficit Disorder, or Personality Disorder.

Not only that, but over the course of the last century, society seems to really fill up our plates with responsibilities. You might feel a lot of parental pressure to get good grades or to take certain AP classes. You might engage in rigorous and time-consuming extracurricular activities or even do volunteer work like tutoring younger students. Maybe you're beginning your college applications or working on your GED.

You've got a lot going on, and it doesn't help anxiety.

Social media can also play a role in the development of anxiety. If you scroll through post after post of your peers in graduation gowns with tons of honors cords or friends wearing expensive clothing, it's difficult to feel like you'll measure up.

It's okay to feel that way for a while, but managing your anxiety and mitigating it as much as possible is important to maintaining a positive self-image.

Managing Anxiety

It's possible to manage your anxiety and live a healthy, happy life. If you feel you may suffer from anxiety, please reach out to a provider or mental health professional.

It's also important to take matters into your own hands. There are many steps you can take to help yourself overcome your anxiety. Let's explore.

Improving your physical health can mitigate symptoms of anxiety. You've heard it before — eat healthy, colorful meals, avoid excessive caffeine and alcohol, get physical activity, etc. You know this already and you have the tools to take these steps. Try taking a brief walk outside and think about your feelings. Really dig into the "why." Use this time to reflect on your life and how you treat your body.

Try practicing mindfulness. Mindfulness is the habit of living in the moment. It involves careful reflection on what you are doing and why you might do it. While you're spending time with friends, focus on your actions and words at that moment. We can only control what's directly in front of us.

Try to avoid thinking of the next thing. While you're with friends, think about what you're feeling and doing. Don't think about assignments due tomorrow or a fight you had with your sibling. Practicing mindfulness is a powerful tool that affects your entire outlook.

Avoid procrastination. I know it's hard. It's tempting to tell yourself, "Well, I can do that assignment the day before," or, "I don't have to try that hard in practice today; I'll just work harder next week." It's hard to tackle assignments and tasks when they aren't looking at you directly. But this is a dangerous game to play. Think about the last time you procrastinated. Your teacher assigned a project to be due next week. You received the rubric and expectations, but you tuck the paper into the back of your folder and move on with the day. You can do it later, right?

The night before the project is due comes much sooner than you'd expected. You panic and scramble to find the rubric and quickly text friends to see if they've completed it. You don't want to cheat, but you need help. It's a huge project.

You feel upset, concerned, and worried. You might even feel a tinge of self-blame because you got yourself into this mess. So, you scramble to complete the project, but it's not your best work and you turn it in feeling dejected. You get your grade back and it's not what you'd hoped.

Procrastination fuels anxiety. It sets you up for failure. Tackle your assignments and tasks head-on. Do them in chunks and review what you've already completed.

Make your anxiety work for you.

Depression

Scrap what you think you know about depression. Depression doesn't look a certain way. It may not involve isolation, suicidal ideation, or neglecting certain tasks. This mindset can be dangerous. Those suffering from depression wear many hats. Oftentimes, they might seem perfectly happy.

Depression comes in many forms, but it is characterized under the umbrella of mood disorders. Depression sometimes involves major depressive episodes that last for months or even years, but it can also last a shorter time, just a few weeks. Some people suffering from depression experience periods where they feel perfectly fine, but suddenly find themselves experiencing feelings of hopelessness. These episodes often happen without any cause or warning, but it's important to understand the different ways depression may develop.

The symptoms of depression might be hard to spot. People with depression can put on a "mask" to avoid confrontation or work through the issue (Smith et al., 2018). It's also important to note that teens and adults experience depression differently.

I suffered from depression throughout my teens and early twenties. I was one of the "maskers," and I worked hard to hide my feelings. On the outside, I took part in sports, volunteer work, and other activities. In my twenties, I joined a sorority and served as a member of our executive board. No one knew what I was feeling, which only made me feel more isolated.

When I did share my struggle, those around me didn't believe it. I remember my father saying, "You don't look depressed."

But I was. Depression is experienced differently and comes in many shapes and sizes. Treat those around you with sensitivity. We never know what other people are going through.

Symptoms of depression in teenagers include the following.

- persistent negativity
- troubles at school or work
- loss of interest in friends or activities
- drug and alcohol abuse
- reckless behavior
- low self-esteem
- sensitivity to criticism
- irritability
- suicidal ideation
- brain fog or lack of mental clarity

It's important to address depression as early as possible.

Just like anxiety, depression can snowball. When the sufferer begins to step away from friends and family, they can experience low self-esteem or feelings of worthlessness. These feelings might lead them to drink alcohol or abuse certain drugs. And these behaviors may lead them to experience thoughts of suicide.

Suicidal ideation is very serious and should be treated as such. If you notice a friend joking about suicide, even in a small way, take notice. If you find yourself saying things like, "I wish I were gone," take action. Suicide is no joking matter. If you're experiencing suicidal thoughts, reach out to a professional or text the National Crisis Textline for help.

It's important to treat depression and acknowledge your struggle. We'll cover specific treatment options later in this section, but for now, know that you're not alone. You don't deserve to feel this way. No one does.

Causes of Depression

Like anxiety, depression can have both environmental and genetic causes. If your mother or sister suffers from depression, it's likely you might as well.

Common environmental and situational causes of depression include being bullied by peers or family, stressful experiences and PTSD, and a lack of social support. But these aren't the only external causes of depression. Assault, anxiety, rejection, or financial difficulties can cause depression in teens and young adults.

If you notice a friend struggling with self-image or bullying, reach out to them. Offer your support. No one deserves to suffer alone.

Treatments

Luckily, there are many treatment options for those suffering from depression. Remember to always consult a medical or mental health professional before trying any of the options we discuss.

Cognitive Behavioral Therapy

The most common treatment method for those suffering from depression is Cognitive Behavioral Therapy, otherwise known as CBT. CBT involves examining problems at their source and rationalizing our reactions. CBT helps the sufferer understand why they feel a certain way and allows them to process their reality through a different lens (Smith et al., 2019).

Interpersonal Therapy

Interpersonal therapy is another treatment method for depression. Interpersonal therapy helps the individual understand the importance of healthy boundaries and relationships. Setting healthy boundaries and surrounding yourself with those who support you is important to guide your recovery.

Medications

Medication is another common tool to manage depression. Your provider may prescribe you medication if your symptoms become moderate to severe. Don't be afraid. Antidepressants and mood-stabilizing medications won't change who you are as a person. Medication has come a long way and will help you manage your day-to-day tasks and help you toward recovery.

Your medical professional may ask you to adopt healthier behaviors as well. Eating healthy foods and exercising can increase the chemicals in your brain that make you feel happy. Listen to your body and pay attention to how you feel.

Depression is a potentially dangerous and sometimes a life-threatening condition. You don't deserve to suffer.

Take steps to improve your mental health, and don't be afraid to ask for help.

An Overview of Mental Illness

Depression and anxiety disorders are simply a few of many mental health conditions. Other disorders, like personality disorders (including Borderline Personality Disorder and Histrionic Personality Disorder), Obsessive Compulsive Disorder

(OCD), and Post Traumatic Stress Disorder (PTSD), are just as dangerous and should be acknowledged.

It's worth reiterating that your feelings matter and should be addressed.

There are a wide variety of resources available to those suffering from mental illness. Speak to a parent, guardian, school counselor, trusted teacher, medical provider, or trusted adult if you feel you're experiencing mental illness. If you feel uncomfortable doing so, don't hesitate to reach out to the National Crisis Textline or another call center to seek help.

You don't deserve to suffer alone.

Sexual Harassment

One in three teenage girls in the United States are victims of sexual harassment at the hands of a friend, peer, online predator, or even a family member ("One-Third of Teenage Girls Sexually Harassed Online," 2017). If you find yourself in this category, know that you're not alone. Always remember that you don't deserve to be sexually harassed.

Sexual harassment is defined as unwelcome physical or verbal behavior in a sexual context. Sexual harassment comes in many forms. Some teens find themselves the victim of sexual harassment on the internet, while others may suffer sexual harassment from teachers, peers, or family members.

Sexual harassment via the internet is dangerous and may come with potentially life-changing effects. Online sexual harassment comes in many forms. You might experience lewd or overtly sexual comments on Snapchat or Instagram. Some teens experience sexual gossip or "leaked" photos. This is not okay, and is, in fact, illegal.

Sexual harassment in person is sometimes easier to identify but is just as dangerous. It may look like sexual comments or "jokes" from family members. It could also look like inappropriate touching from a peer or teacher. Additionally, sexual harassment may involve comments about sexual behaviors.

Remember, this is not okay, and you didn't deserve it.

You might be the victim of sexual harassment and not even know it. Sometimes, when we live in an environment that normalizes dangerous sexual behavior, we might see it as simply a part of life.

It is not.

Effects of Sexual Harassment

Sexual harassment doesn't stop after they make the comment. Victims of sexual harassment experience negative long-term effects, including depression, anxiety, eating disorders, insomnia, and poor academic performance.

It's hard to focus on your algebra exam if you're anxious about sexual comments made by your peers between classes.

It's difficult to feel good about your body if you receive scary and inappropriate comments about your appearance from people online.

If you experience these signs of sexual harassment or notice a friend struggling, don't hesitate to reach out for help.

Victims of sexual harassment often feel as though it's their fault, or feel as though they did something to provoke the action. They did not. There is no reason you should be harassed in any manner, especially a sexual one.

We have to stop sexual harassment in its tracks. In some cases, sexual harassment can become sexual violence.

Remember this — you did *nothing* to cause what happened. You didn't deserve this.

Battling Sexual Harassment

Many victims of sexual harassment feel embarrassed, watched, and afraid. You might be afraid to speak up for any of the following reasons.

- worry that nothing will be done to stop the action
- fear of being labeled a "snitch"
- relationship to the harasser
- fear of parental involvement

These are just a few of the reasons many incidents of sexual harassment go unreported.

It's okay to be scared at first. Standing up is difficult and takes serious bravery. You don't deserve what's happening to you, and those who hurt you should be held accountable.

More importantly, if you notice or witness sexual harassment, speak up. It's up to all of us to stop sexual harassment in its tracks.

Contact the RAINN Sexual Violence hotline or speak to a parent or law enforcement officer if you or someone you know is the victim of sexual harassment. It's illegal, and it's up to us to make it stop.

Confidence and How To Build It

You've heard the phrase, "Confidence is key." And yes, it certainly is. But that phrase alone doesn't make *being* or *feeling* confident any easier.

It's hard to be confident in a world full of uncertainty, doubt, and comparison. Your daily tasks, stress from school or activities, and other societal pressures make confidence difficult.

Think about it in these ways: If you're struggling in math class and can't seem to grasp the material, you might feel a little down or doubtful of your abilities. If you feel you don't look like the women labeled "beautiful" online, you might feel unattractive or unworthy.

It's okay to feel that way for a little while, but confidence is a comprehensive practice. Being confident involves examining the scope of who you are as a person. You can feel uncertain about your singing abilities but confident in your classes. We have to see the whole, not the parts.

I struggled with confidence for the majority of my teens. It's hard, it really is. I was a serial perfectionist. I felt bombarded with responsibilities and tasks; pressure from my parents to attend college and get good grades didn't help.

Some advice? Fake it. Fake confidence. Walk tall and walk proudly. Act unapologetically to you. Pretend you love everything about yourself. If you act confident, others will think you are.

And over time, you'll feel confident all on your own.

Puberty and Confidence

Think about how you felt about yourself before entering puberty. You probably didn't think much of the way your body looked or the color of your hair. You were simply you.

Puberty is a time of drastic physical and mental change. It's when you become a woman. Parts of your body are growing in ways you don't understand and don't know what to do with. It's a little scary. It's okay to be afraid of the unknown.

In general, sometime around the age of twelve, girls tend to experience lower confidence than their male counterparts do (Shipman et al., 2018). Psychologists believe it has to do with rumination or a preoccupation with certain negative feelings. When we're bombarded with negative thoughts and piles of responsibilities, we feel worse about ourselves.

Typically, teenage girls take fewer risks and engage in fewer risky behaviors than their guy friends and peers, which could cause lower confidence as well.

And let's be real. Our responsibilities really pile up after puberty. After puberty, we build up a laundry list of things we absolutely positively *have* to do. You might have to look a certain way before leaving for school. When you arrive there, you have tests and exams and problem sets. You think it's important for you to do well on them to reach your future goals and make your parents proud. You go to theater auditions and shoot for the lead role in that year's spring musical. Then you arrive home and take quizzes, finish homework, and clean your room. Maybe you have to make dinner or do the laundry on top of all that.

Girl, it's a lot.

This pressure negatively affects our self-confidence.

I'm not asking you to forget your homework or neglect your chores; I'm asking you to examine your life from a bird's eye view. Don't be too hard on yourself.

Building Confidence

With all that being said, it's important to know how to build your own confidence. You deserve to feel good about yourself, no matter what! Let's talk about a few of the ways you can increase your confidence and accomplish your big-girl goals.

Achievement Lists

Begin by writing out your achievements. Literally, make a list. This list can look just like the one we did in the last chapter, but try to focus on concrete achievements. Maybe you earned an A on a particularly difficult essay. Maybe you scored that lead role in the spring musical or made a killer plate of spaghetti.

Add to the list over time. Pull it out when you feel down. There are things about you that are really cool and admirable. We can't expect others to think we're great unless we do first.

Befriend Failure

Learn to accept failure. Ivy League students fail tests. Thomas Edison made thousands of lightbulbs that simply didn't turn on. Olympic athletes don't win every race.

Failure is a part of life, and it's certainly an important one. Think about the last time you "failed." It might've been a test or project. Maybe you failed a friend in need. Perhaps you forgot to do an important chore or a personal task.

Instead of dwelling on what happened, think about it as a learning experience. We learn more from failures than we do from successes.

If you fail an important essay, look at the margins and read the teacher's comments. They're probably making some good points. Use those points to better your next essay and you might do better.

Apply that mindset to the rest of your life. Failure is universal. I've failed many times. But I learned from my failures. I adapted and grew from setbacks.

You can do it too.

Stand Up For Yourself

This one is pretty tricky if you're like me and struggle to stand up to authority figures; it's daunting.

I feared teachers, coaches, family friends, and even my dad. I'd cower and my heart would race after a class or meeting. It was terrifying.

Standing up for yourself doesn't mean you have to be rude or bossy; it involves acknowledging when something is unfair or unjust and pointing it out.

Let's say your coach said something you feel crossed the line in practice. Maybe he said something like, "_____ has the worst form I've ever seen," or, "You throw like a girl," in front of your peers.

What he said wasn't okay. You could let it nag at your confidence and trigger self-doubt, or you could address the problem at its core.

You choose the latter.

You ask him for a moment of his time and explain why you

felt uncomfortable with what he said. If he had a problem with your form or throwing, he should've brought it to your attention in private.

You might be thinking, "What if he doesn't do what I ask?" or, "Will he think less of me?"

These thoughts are perfectly valid.

Think about it this way: If he doesn't do what you ask and cut the comments, you can address him again. You could get a parent or guardian involved.

What I do know is that he won't think less of you; in fact, he'll respect you for standing up for yourself and setting boundaries.

You deserve to feel heard.

Change Your Language

Look back at the last few sections. Think about the language I used. Our language is a direct result of how we think about ourselves and the world around us. Changing our language is a powerful step toward changing our mindset.

When I discussed achievements, I used the word "earn," not the word "got." You worked hard to achieve what you have, so acknowledge that. Instead of saying "mistake," call it a setback. A mistake means something negative, while a setback has a better connotation.

Language extends to what you say or don't say. Instead of saying, "Gosh, my hair is so frizzy today," say, "You know, I think this outfit is really working." Instead of saying, "That class is so freaking hard," say, "Algebra is really challenging right now."

Speak to yourself in a positive way. Don't harass yourself or break yourself down over minor setbacks. Other people do that enough. You have to befriend yourself to gain confidence. You deserve to feel good.

Period Pennings

We've learned a lot, and this was a pretty heavy chapter. Use these questions to breathe and reflect on what you've learned. Your mental health is just as important as your physical health, so treat it that way! Stand up for yourself and set boundaries.

It's okay to struggle, and it's okay to feel unworthy. But you alone have the power to change how you feel.

Fill in the blanks below to reflect on your own mental health.

- Sometimes I feel _____and _____about my mental health.
- I struggle with _____, so I will reach out to _____ and _____ to get support.
- I noticed _____ today, and I plan to do _____to change it.
- _____ is happening to me or someone I know. I want to do _____and _____ to help them and myself.
- I achieved _____ recently, and I felt _____ about it.
- I want to improve my confidence and I plan to try _____, _____, and _____to better myself.

Chapter 6: Oh, I Am What I Am

So, what is gender identity? Well, it's complicated. Gender identity refers to your sense of who you are and what gender you identify with. You might identify as male, female, gender neutral, transgender, or non-binary. Your gender identity is an important part of who you are.

Before we continue, I want to identify and explain a few terms I'll refer to when discussing gender identity. It's important to be aware of the language we use when talking about gender.

The term **cisgender** refers to someone who identifies with the gender they were given at birth.

The term **transgender** refers to those who feel their gender identity does not align with the gender they were given at birth. Transgender people may take steps to alter their gender.

Gender fluid refers to those who experience transience when it comes to their gender identity. They may feel they identify as a female sometimes and male at other times. They might experience periods where they don't identify as either.

Non-binary refers to individuals who feel their gender identity doesn't fit in a specific category. In other words, they don't identify as explicitly male or female and feel their gender is separate from these two terms.

Agender refers to people who don't feel they have a specific gender. Agender and non-binary are different terms; those who identify as non-binary feel they're a blend of male and female, while those who identify as agender feel they do not or cannot fit in either category.

I also want to note that gender identity has nothing to do with sexual identity. Someone who is transgender may also identify as gay or straight; the two are not related.

Think about your own gender identity. Do you feel you're cisgender or transgender? Maybe you don't feel like you fit in any category at all. That's okay. There are many resources to help you figure it out!

Gender Development

We begin expressing our gender identity when we're around two or three years old. Children this age are aware of the differences between men and women, but mostly on a surface level; they notice boys wear different clothing than girls and they can probably understand how they act differently. Two and three-year-olds might express their gender through playing with certain toys and clothing, or engaging in certain activities.

Between the ages of four to seven, children begin to gain a stable idea of their gender identity. Girls who feel confident in their gender identity might enjoy wearing bright pink dresses and Disney-themed shoes. I was a big fan of brightly colored Bermuda shorts. Younger children who feel unsure of their gender might feel social anxiety around others and reject certain activities.

As a teenager, you might have a good idea of how you identify in terms of your gender. Our gender identity is affected by personal, mental, and environmental factors. Teens may experiment with different styles or languages to identify who they are.

Puberty is an important time for both those confident and unsure of their gender identity. People who identify as cisgender may feel more confident in their changing body, whereas those who feel they might identify differently might be upset or anxious.

If you feel you fall into this category, you're not alone! Many young people (and older people) struggle with their gender identity.

It's important to remember that your interest, style, activities, or sports don't determine your gender identity. Liking dark pants and video games doesn't mean you're a boy, it means you like those things.

You determine your gender identity for yourself.

Gender Dysphoria

Gender dysphoria refers to when you feel your gender identity doesn't align with the one you were given at birth. Don't be scared! Many people experience gender dysphoria.

Gender dysphoria and identifying as transgender are two different things. You might struggle with gender dysphoria but find you're agender, non-binary, or gender fluid.

Those with gender dysphoria may display the following signs.

- anxiety when engaging with others or in certain social situations
- growing upset when others identify you a certain way
- ask to be referred to by pronouns that don't align with the ones they were given at birth

- ask questions about their gender and what it means for their body

Gender dysphoria requires a medical diagnosis, but having gender dysphoria doesn't mean you're mentally ill. The term refers to those who experience stress about their gender identity, which often leads the individual to take steps to change it.

Doctors use the following criteria to diagnose gender dysphoria.

- expressing the desire to get rid of one's gendered traits for a period longer than six months
- desire to be another gender, which includes nonbinary, gender fluid, or agender
- a need to be treated as the gender they wish to assume
- feeling as though you experience thoughts that align with those of another gender identity

Don't use these metrics to diagnose yourself. Seek a medical professional if you experience these symptoms.

If you feel you're experiencing gender dysphoria, know that you're not alone. Many people struggle to identify their gender and may feel a degree of discomfort at expressing their feelings. There are many resources available to you, and we'll discuss those later in the chapter.

Gender Expression

We express our gender in a wide variety of ways. If you identify as female (whether that be cisgender-female or transgender-female) you might express your femininity through clothing choices or hairstyles. You might choose to go by a traditionally female nickname or you might engage in certain activities that align with your gender identity.

If you identify differently, you might try to find clothing, styles, or activities that align with your gender identity. You may avoid certain clothing or hairstyles to express how you feel about your gender. You may also use pronouns that align with how you feel.

At first, those who identify differently than the gender they were assigned at birth dive into styles they feel identify them. Thosewho feel they're transgender may rush to get a haircut or throw out the pink in their closet. You might not do this at all.

Gender expression and gender identity are completely different. Disliking skirts and dresses and preferring pants or darker colors doesn't determine your gender identity.

Gender expression refers to the way you like to express your gender. We all have different preferences and styles, so choose a style that makes you feel comfortable.

You Feel Confused About Your Gender Identity: What's Next?

It's okay to feel confused if the way you express your gender doesn't align with the gender you were assigned at birth. That's okay and normal. This doesn't mean you have gender dysphoria.

Gender dysphoria and breaking traditional gender norms about expression are different. I identify as female and hate skirts and the color pink. Those who identify as male can wear earrings or paint their nails and still identify as male.

Express yourself how you please!

If you feel confused about how you identify, that's okay. You're certainly not alone. Many teens feel apprehensive about seeking help or taking the next steps to determine their gender identity, so let's discuss.

Gender Discomfort

It's okay to feel a bit uncomfortable when exploring your gender identity.

If you feel you don't identify as cisgender and feel you have gender dysphoria, you might "feel a strong sense of being a gender that is different to the sex you were assigned at birth and may feel that this has affected the way you feel about your body" (*Worried About Your Gender Identity? Advice for Teenagers,* 2022).

Remember, gender identity issues aren't a mental illness. You don't have a disease and it's normal to struggle to identify your gender. But that doesn't make it more comfortable.

Those struggling with gender discomfort might feel a lot of

stress when socializing and can even experience low academic performance. Some people struggling with gender discomfort might experience depression or anxiety, which negatively affects their ability to participate in certain activities.

It doesn't have to be this way.

So what do you do next? Luckily, you have many options.

How to Get Help

Help for those working through gender dysphoria is plentiful, and there are many resources available to you.

The first step to getting help is talking to a trusted adult. This can be a family member or family friend. If you don't feel comfortable discussing this with them for any reason, try speaking to a trusted teacher, professor, or school counselor.

If you don't feel comfortable with those options, that's okay. The adults in your life may have differing opinions about how you choose to identify, and that's on them.

Most communities have many gender identity support groups. If you can't find one in your area, there are many support groups that meet online or via Zoom, allowing you to attend without transportation.

The next step is learning about your options. Examine what you want and what you feel is your gender identity. There are many agencies around the world designed to help you understand these options and put them into action.

I'll focus on the Gender Identity Development Service, or GIDS, as an example. Remember, there are other options; we just have to Google them.

GIDS, as well as many other agencies, begin with a detailed assessment of you and your environment. This involves an examination of your current gender identity, as well as gender identities you've assumed in the past.

This assessment will help them gauge your needs and options. You might be referred to a mental health professional who can help you talk through some of your concerns and discomforts. Like I said before, identifying differently does not make you mentally ill. It's okay to struggle, and there are professionals who can help you navigate your gender journey.

If you feel you'd like to take the next steps to change your gender identity, you may be referred to hormone therapy. Hormone therapy can involve different options, including hormone blockers that prolong puberty or taking male or female sex hormones to change your gender identity over time.

Hormone therapy can affect your fertility, so it's important to consider these options carefully. It's not meant to be scary, but it is a big decision. Use the resources around you to help you make an educated choice.

The Future of Your Gender

Like I said, it's not meant to be scary, but it is okay to be nervous. Your gender identity is yours and yours alone. You might feel a lot of pressure to be a certain way, act a certain way, or look a certain way, but ultimately you have the choice to choose how you identify.

Don't let society tell you how to express your gender. Society gets it wrong sometimes. You're your own baddie, no matter how you identify.

If you feel uncomfortable in your gender identity or feel you're experiencing gender dysphoria, please seek the resources I provide. There is always help around you; we just have to know where to look.

Period Pennings

I hope this chapter taught you more about how gender works and how you can express or change your gender identity. Everyone deserves to feel comfy in their own skin, and you choose how to identify.

Use these questions and fill in the answers to explore what you know about gender and how you feel about your own.

It's okay to be honest, no one has to know what you've written but you!

- I feel _____ about my current gender identity.
- I currently express my gender identity through my _____, my_____, and my _____.
- I want to _____ my gender identity.
- Growing up, I felt _____ about the way I identify myself.
- I think trying _____ and _____ to express my gender identity might be cool.

Chapter 7: I like Who I Like

Sexuality isn't just sex. Sexuality refers to who you like and how you like them.

Like I said in the last chapter, sexual orientation and gender identity are entirely different; sexuality, or sexual orientation, involves who you're attracted to in a sexual and romantic way.

But sexuality can be a little more complicated than that. Many people, maybe even yourself, may struggle to understand their sexual orientation, and media outlets don't always help.

In this chapter, we'll discuss the factors contributing to your sexuality, as well as its role in our media. It's okay to feel a little confused. We'll talk about it!

Sexuality In Popular Culture

Think about the pop culture icons you love; the Kardashians, TikTok stars, etc. Do they talk openly about their sexuality?

Many do!

Conversations about sexuality and sexual orientation are becoming increasingly normalized thanks to popular culture and societal change. In fact, the "more heavily pop culture incorporates sexuality the less sensitive society becomes" (Trew,

2o11).

Many celebrities are viewed as role models for the gay community, including Madonna, Elton John, Fergie, Miley Cyrus, and Lady Gaga.

It's great there are so many openly gay celebrities, but it's not all glitz, glamour, and pride flags.

Pop culture's "overuse of sexuality as a marketing tool also makes this very influence an area of great concern" (Trew, 2011). Pop culture has a tendency to oversexualize those who identify as non-heterosexual, which leads to damaging misconceptions about sexuality and how to express it.

Remember, your sexual identity isn't your *entire* identity. It's simply a very small part of who you are.

Pop culture's emphasis on sexuality can cause teens to feel pressure to be "sexually active earlier, to be worried about body image well before the body has finished developing, [and] to value sexuality before other aspects of life" (Trew, 2011).

TV shows, movies, and TikTok stars can emphasize a certain lifestyle that hinges on their sexuality. While sexuality is important to becoming who you are, it isn't the be-all-end-all.

Sex is important to our culture, and discussions about sexuality should praise and respect how people identify. Unfortunately, pressure from mass media to sensationalize sexuality can have an adverse effect and can cause teens to value their sexuality and sexual identity in misguided ways.

It's great that these discussions are more normalized than they were in the past. Providing a space for people to openly discuss sexuality and sexual orientation is empowering.

Remember that you're more than who you do or don't have sex with. We describe our identity and personality through many different adjectives and nouns, and gay, straight, or bisexual are only a few of them.

Your Crash Course Into Sexual Orientation

There are many ways you may choose to sexually identify.

It's important to understand that all of your feelings are completely normal and valid.

Sexual identity doesn't refer to only sex. In fact, sexual identity is more about intimacy, attraction, and how to develop and maintain healthy relationships.

Keep in mind that "gay" isn't a no-no word and shouldn't be used as an insult. It's the same as saying, "you run like a girl." Embrace your sexuality, regardless of the word.

Remember that sexuality exists on a spectrum. No one is explicitly straight or explicitly gay. Your sexuality may even change over time!

Let's talk about the different terms used to identify one's sexual orientation.

Heterosexual refers to those attracted to members of the opposite sex. If you identify as a heterosexual female, you would be attracted to those who identify as male.

Homosexual refers to those attracted to members of the same sex. So, for instance, if you identify as a homosexual female, you would be attracted to other women.

Bisexual refers to people attracted to members of both sexes. Those who identify as a biscxual female would be attracted to both women and men.

Pansexual refers to those attracted to all genders, regardless of the other person's gender identity. Pansexuality and bisexuality are different. Those who identify as pansexual may be attracted to someone who identifies as gender-fluid or gender-neutral, while someone who is bisexual is attracted to both men and women.

Demisexual is a relatively new term used to identify those who only experience sexual attraction if they feel an emotional connection with another person. For example, if you identify as demisexual, you would only feel attracted to another classmate if you liked them or were in a relationship with them. It's possible to identify as both demisexual and heterosexual, homosexual, pansexual, or bisexual.

Asexual refers to those who do not feel a sexual attraction towards members of any gender identification.

You've probably heard of Lesbian, Gay, Bisexual, Transgender, and Questioning (LGBTQ); the term LGBTQ is used by those who fit into the above categories to identify themselves.

How Do I Know How I Identify?

Well, it gets a bit tricky. If you feel you might identify with certain sexuality, especially if it's not heterosexuality, you might be a little confused or anxious.

Here are some signs you might identify differently.

- You have fantasies or dreams about sex with members of different genders.
- You feel confused or anxious when discussing sex.
- You feel upset in certain situations when sex is being discussed.
- You feel differently about your sexuality after a consensual sexual encounter.

Uncertainty stinks.

It's quite common to feel unsure about how you identify sexually, and many external factors and pressures don't help.

Some people experiencing confusion or uncertainty regarding their sexual orientation may experience a fear of social stigmas surrounding sexual identity, fear of rejection or lack of acceptance by friends or family, or a lack of knowledge regarding sexuality (*Teenage sexuality*, 2021).

Consider how you feel about your sexuality, especially if you identify with any of the signs or fears discussed earlier. It's okay to feel different from your peers.

In fact, if you're questioning your sexuality, you fit into the "Q" part of LGBTQ!

What Causes Sexual Orientation?

Biology! Sexual orientation is genetic and is determined before birth, so it's impossible to "turn gay" or "turn straight." Many people feel attracted to a certain gender before puberty; for others, it might take a little longer to discover their sexual orientation.

But sexuality isn't necessarily set. Your sexuality can change throughout the course of your life.

Our lives are filled with rich experiences and reactions to what we see and do. You might feel you identify a certain way, only to feel differently after watching a TV show or movie.

Again, these reactions didn't "turn" you a certain way. They helped you realize who you are and how you identify.

Feeling Alone?

You're not. Many people identify as members of the LGBTQ community. About 11% of adults in the United States admit they feel some attraction to members of the same gender, and 8.2% of adults report they've experienced a sexual encounter with a member of the same sex (*What causes sexual orientation?*, n.d.).

But this varies from region to region. In some parts of the U.S., like San Francisco or New York City, this percentage is much higher.

It's also important to note that this percentage has risen over the past fifty years. For a long time, sexuality was a taboo topic, and members of the LGBTQ community felt a strong pressure to live a heterosexual life.

We live in an exciting age of change and acceptance. Embrace it!

Can people "tell" how I sexually identify?

Nope, not at all. At least, not until you tell them. Other people might think they know your sexual orientation (think about the term "gaydar"), but this is simply a misconception.

Just because you dress a certain way or engage in certain sports does not mean you identify as gay, straight, bisexual, or pansexual. I played a lot of video games in my teens, but I didn't identify as gay, regardless of what those around me believed.

Sexual orientation is a personal decision and doesn't have any bearing on how you identify your gender.

Teenage Sexuality

You might have questions about sexuality and what it means for you; that's perfectly normal! It's common to have questions or different understandings of sexuality, especially as a pre-teen or teenager. Your body is growing in new ways and you're beginning to discover your sexual identity.

It's pretty exciting!

We established how your brain changes during puberty in chapters one and two. But it doesn't stop at sleep: your brain changes emotionally and physiologically during puberty.

These new emotions play a role in your budding sexuality. You might begin to experience sexual attraction to people in your math class or you might simply want to be closer to a friend you met in softball club. Maybe there's someone in your English class who's especially funny.

You might want to feel drawn to sexual activity. You might not, and that's also okay.

Facing the choice to be sexually active is an important part of the growing-up process, regardless of your feelings. There is no "right age" to become sexually active. You get to decide when the right time is for you and a consenting partner.

Sexual Activity

When most people think about the word sex, they think of vaginal intercourse, but there are many ways you can communicate your love or affection to a partner regardless of your sexual orientation.

Kissing or spending time with another person is one way to express your feelings physically, as is touching or oral sex (Paul,

2020).

It's important to understand your options so you can make educated decisions about what you are and aren't comfortable with. I'm by no means saying you should do or try everything I discuss here; you should understand what sexual intercourse often entails so you can become an informed adult.

Information is better than no information, right?

You might feel uncomfortable discussing sex, and you might even feel uncomfortable reading about it. That's okay! New things are uncomfortable. If you feel uncomfortable reading the material in this section, take a step back and rationalize how you feel.

Touching another person in a sexual context involves touching their sexual organs. Certain parts of our bodies are sensitive to stimulation, and sexual touching stimulates those areas.

Oral sex involves stimulating these areas with your mouth. Either party, regardless of gender, can engage in oral sex.

Anal sex is often associated with members of the LGBTQ community, but that's a misconception. Anal sex involves penetrating the anus, which can be done by either consenting party.

Vaginal intercourse is most often associated with sex. It involves penetrating the consenting person's vagina with a male sex organ or another object.

Masturbation is also a part of sex. Masturbation is often considered taboo, especially for young women, but it's not meant to be! Masturbation is an empowering way to discover your own body by touching yourself in stimulating areas. It's a sort of trial run: you learn what you like and don't like!

Your decision to participate in any or none of these activities is up to you. You have the right to choose when you engage in sex.

It's your choice, which brings us to consent.

Consent

Consent means you or the other party enthusiastically agree to what's happening between you and it's a key part of healthy, positive sex.

Asking for consent might feel uncomfortable at first, but it's very important. You want someone to want you, right?

And more importantly, you have the right to say yes or no to what's happening.

Remember, someone who is under the influence cannot give consent, even if they say yes. This is similarly a form of sexual assault.

You have the right to revoke your consent at any time. If you feel uncomfortable with what's happening, you can speak up. Just because you gave your partner permission in the past, doesn't mean you can't say no in the future.

You have the right to what happens to your body, and you make the choice.

If someone does something to you without your consent, it's not your fault. Please seek resources or talk to a trusted adult if this happens. You did nothing wrong and you deserve consent.

Talking About Sexuality

Discussing your sexuality isn't easy, especially when you feel "out of the norm." Remember, you're not alone. You don't have to share everything at once, nor do you have to share anything at all. Talking about your sexuality with those around you can be a powerful tool to accept it, but this is your conversation. You have control.

Begin by telling one person first. Don't group people together if you aren't comfortable doing so.

If you have someone around you, whether it be a parent, friend, trusted adult, or counselor, begin sharing with them. If you have reservations about how they might react, choose someone else!

It might be a good idea to seek an adult or friend who's open about their sexuality. If you know someone who identifies as a member of the LGBTQ community, reach out to them. If not, there are many call and text centers that are more than happy to guide you through this process.

Understand that we cannot control how others react, but we can control what we share with them. You might feel confident sharing your feelings with someone, only to be met with harsh language or rejection.

It hurts, it really does. It's okay to be upset if this happens, but remember, it's a "them" problem, not a "you" problem. You can't "make" someone feel a certain way. You're not responsible for anyone's feelings, but your own.

Some conversations may be difficult, so be prepared to explain how you feel. Sometimes parents, even those who understand and support members of the LGBTQ community, may have different feelings about your sexuality. It takes time to accept new information. People may not accept you, but again, that's a "them" problem.

Accepting your sexuality is difficult and takes time. You might feel confused, angry, upset, or lost. That's okay and to be expected.

You deserve to honor your feelings, and this includes honoring your sexuality.

After all, you like who you like.

Period Pennings

That was a lot of info, so let's reflect. We learned about sexuality, acceptance, sex, and consent. I hope you gained important information about identifying yourself and honoring your body. You deserve to feel comfortable.

Fill in the blanks to these questions to gauge your understanding and to help you rationalize your feelings:

- My celebrity crush is _____. I think they're so _____!
- When I feel attracted to someone, I tend to look for these qualities: _____, _____, _____, and _____.
- I tend to feel _____ when discussing sexuality.
- I think I identify as _____, but I'm unsure for these reasons: _____, _____, _____.
- I feel drawn to _____ person/people because of _____.

Chapter 8: An Unprotected Mess

Regardless of how you feel about sexual activity, it's important to know all of your options. We discussed your ability to choose in the last chapter. In this chapter, we'll talk about the importance of educating yourself about your options and how to protect yourself when engaging in sexual activity.

Let's talk about what happens before and after sex.

Teen Sex Stats

Many people in the United States begin exploring sex during their teen years. In fact, a study conducted by the Center for Disease Control (CDC) found that about 40% of teens, both male and female, are sexually active or have engaged in the act of sexual activity (Abma & Martinez, 2019). The percentage is slightly higher for male teenagers.

Let's break it down by age. Many teens begin experimenting with sex around the age of fifteen or sixteen, but men seem to begin experimenting a bit earlier than women.

Before age fifteen, 16% of male teens and 11% of female teens report having had sexual intercourse (Abma & Martinez, 2019).

As teens get older, the percentage increases. By age eighteen, 55% of both male and female teens report having had sexual intercourse (Abma & Martinez, 2019).

It also seems that the nature of the relationship between sexual partners plays a role in one's choice to engage in sexual activity. Both female and male teens are more likely to have sexual intercourse with a romantic partner, but male teenagers report a higher rate of sexual intercourse with someone they'd call a friend.

Contraceptive use has drastically increased in recent years; teens are much more likely to protect themselves, which is great! It seems that the younger one begins to experiment with sexual activity, the less likely they are to use contraception.

Overall, 81% of teens between the ages of fifteen and eighteen report using contraception in some form the first time they engage in sexual intercourse (Abma & Martinez, 2019).

81% is a vast improvement, but the percentage still isn't perfect.

In most classes, an 81% would be a B-.

It's important that members of all sexes understand how to protect themselves, regardless of sexual orientation or gender identity.

Let's discuss safe sex practices and the dangers of unsafe sex. Remember, you deserve to know your options.

Sexual Health

Sexual health is defined as "a state of physical, emotional, mental, and social well-being in relation to sexuality" (*11 facts about sexual health in teens in the US*, 2015).

Sexual health is deeply intertwined with physical health.

Unsafe sexual habits can lead to unwanted diseases or even pregnancy.

Remember, it's your choice whether or not to engage in sexual activity. There is no "right" age to begin, and the choice is up to you.

Let's talk about some ways you can protect yourself when engaging in sexual intercourse.

Condoms

They're cheap, easy to use, and widely available. They're the most common form of contraception among teenagers and can be used by anyone regardless of gender or sexual orientation.

Condoms are readily available at supermarkets, gas stations, and some schools or health clinics have them for free or at low prices.

Condoms are the easiest way to protect yourself from Sexually Transmitted Diseases (STDs) because they create a barrier between you and your partner, blocking the infection from being transmitted.

Not only that, condoms are an effective way to protect against pregnancy. They can be combined with other methods of birth control to be even more effective.

Prescription Birth Control

Prescription birth control is just that — birth control you get from a medical professional. It's important to know that prescription birth control only protects against pregnancy, not against STDs.

There are various types of prescription birth control methods, and we'll discuss a few here.

Always speak to a medical professional before trying any of these methods. Learn about your options before choosing what's best for you and your body.

The "Pill"

The pill is the most common birth control method among teens and adults. The pill works in a variety of ways, depending on the type of pill you're prescribed. In most cases, the pill works by "stopping ovulation (the release of an egg from an ovary), thickening cervical mucus to keep sperm from entering the uterus, [or] thinning the lining of the uterus so that a fertilized egg is less likely to attach" (*Birth control pill: contraception, the till, effectiveness, types*, 2020).

The pill takes about seven days to begin working, so plan accordingly.

There are many pros of the pill; teens report experiencing lighter periods and improvement in acne. Certain pills can lower the risk of cancer (*Birth Control Pill: Contraception, the Pill, Effectiveness, Types,* 2020). The cons of the pill are that some women experience side effects like breast tenderness.

Remember, the pill does not prevent STDs or sexually transmitted diseases.

The IUD

Intrauterine Devices (IUD) is a long-term form of birth control inserted into the uterus by a medical professional.

The IUD is among one of the most "foolproof" forms of birth control and works in two different ways: copper IUDs stop the sperm from fertilizing the egg, whereas hormonal IUDs release hormones that stop ovulation.

IUDs can last longer than other forms of contraception and are available in two-year, five-year, and ten-year forms. The pros of the IUD are that you never have to think about it and they're quite effective when inserted properly. The con is that some women report discomfort when the IUD is inserted and may experience heavier periods.

The Arm Insert

Some women opt for an arm insert. This form of birth control involves inserting a small rod into the arm; this rod releases hormones that prevent pregnancy at its source.

This form of birth control lasts for three years and must be inserted by a medical professional.

The pros of the insert are that it lasts a long time, and usually doesn't cause many side effects. The cons are that it's not as effective as other methods of birth control and can shift if misplaced; and it can be a little scary if you're afraid of needles.

The Shot

This form of birth control has a scary name, but it's not scary at all.

The shot is pretty much just that — quarterly shot that manages your hormones. The shot works in two ways: it prevents ovulation using the hormone progesterone, and thickens the mucus around your cervix, preventing semen from reaching the vagina (*Are there birth control shot side effects?*, n.d.).

It sounds a little gross, but don't fear. It's science.

The pro of the shot is you don't have to think about it too much; it's a pretty self-explanatory form of birth control. The cons are that it can cause side effects like spotting and weight gain (*Are there birth control shot side effects?*, n.d.), and again, it can be a little scary if you're afraid of needles!

You have to make sure to attend your doctor's appointments regularly when relying on the shot. After 12-13 weeks, it won't be nearly as effective.

Takeaways

It's your choice whether or not you decide to use birth control or other forms of contraception. Speak to a doctor or practitioner before trying any of these options.

Make an educated choice for you and your body.

Unsafe Sex

If you choose to engage in sexual activity, you have to know the risks. Contraception can greatly decrease your risk of STDs and pregnancy, but the chances are never zero.

Luckily, there are many ways you can prevent and treat STDs at the source.

STDs are certain diseases or infections that are transmitted through sexual contact. STDs can be transmitted through multiple forms of sexual contact, not just vaginal intercourse. Condoms are the most effective way to prevent the spread of STDs.

So what are the common STDs? Unfortunately, there are many. Left untreated, STDs can lead to many health issues and can even cause infertility.

Chlamydia, gonorrhea, HIV, and syphilis are common STDs but are preventable. Some STDs, namely chlamydia and gonorrhea, go without symptoms, so it's important to get tested at a local clinic or by a doctor regularly when engaging in sexual activity.

However, if you do experience any of the following symptoms, please see a medical professional.

- unusual urination patterns
- bleeding between periods
- lower belly pain
- strong smells

Don't be scared. Many STDs are treatable, including chlamydia, gonorrhea, and syphilis. Early detection is important, so check in with a professional regularly.

Beyond contraception and condoms, how do you protect yourself?

Begin by talking to your partner about STDs. It might feel uncomfortable at first, but being protected is important. If your partner isn't comfortable discussing STDs, you need a new partner.

Use a condom every time you engage in sexual activity. Condoms are the only form of contraception that prevents STDs. They're available in both latex and non-latex varieties, so use them!

Do not have sex while under the influence. It's a bit tempting, I know, but you'll be less likely to make an educated decision while under the influence.

Sex is fun and exciting, but diseases and pregnancy aren't (that is, if you're not ready). You deserve to protect your body.

Even more, you deserve a partner that cares about protecting you.

Teen Pregnancy

By now, you probably have a solid understanding of how pregnancy works. Hopefully, you also understand how to prevent it. Teen pregnancy can be a bit more complicated than adult pregnancy and comes with a higher chance of risks to the mother and the baby.

Complications, Risks, and Causes

What are the risks of teen pregnancy? What complications can occur?

The short answer? Too many.

Teenage mothers have a higher likelihood of delivering underweight or malnourished babies, often due to a lack of adequate prenatal care. Babies born to teenage mothers may suffer long-term physical or mental deficits and may be born premature (Adhikari, 2019).

But what about the mothers?

Teenage mothers are much more likely to suffer serious complications through pregnancy, including pre-eclampsia (high blood pressure during pregnancy) and anemia.

Teenage mothers are more likely to drop out of school, suffer unemployment, and experience lower academic performance than their peers.

In the United States, one in four teenage girls becomes pregnant every year (Adhikari, 2019). That's a pretty high number, right? It's likely someone around you has become pregnant, and it's even more likely you don't even know.

So what causes teen pregnancy?

Teen pregnancy is most often caused by the following reasons.

- lack of understanding of protection
- peer pressure
- lack of sex education
- family history of teen pregnancies

We'll discuss more of the causes and misconceptions in the following section. Always remember: education is key.

Misconceptions regarding Teen Pregnancy and Contraception

Teen pregnancy occurs when teens don't understand their options or potential risks. Contraception and birth control are great ways to protect against pregnancy, but oftentimes teens don't understand how to use these correctly.

Unfortunately, there are many other misconceptions regarding what actually causes pregnancy. You can't believe everything you hear.

Let's discuss some of the common misconceptions regarding birth control and safe sex.

Some people use condoms incorrectly. They might seem relatively self-explanatory, but putting a condom on the right way drastically decreases your risk of pregnancy. When using a condom, make sure to push any air through the end to ensure it fits properly. If a condom is too big, it won't be as effective.

Anal sex is *not* an alternative to preventing pregnancy. The odds of becoming pregnant from anal sex are low, but not impossible (Nazario, 2021). Condoms should still be worn while engaging in anal sex.

Having sex during your period can still lead to pregnancy. The odds are lower, but again, not zero. As a teenager, your periods may be irregular, so having unprotected sex while on your period isn't effective without a condom or alternative birth control method.

Contrary to popular belief, you can get pregnant the first time you have sex. Without contraception, sperm always has the opportunity to reach the egg, no matter the timing.

Many teens rely on the pull-out method of birth control to help control pregnancy. Unfortunately, it's not very effective. The pull-out method involves timing one's orgasm and "pulling out" before ejaculation. Sometimes the timing doesn't work, and it's difficult for your partner to understand when they might ejaculate, especially if they're not experienced.

Not only that, but pre-cum (the substance released prior to ejaculation) can also contain semen, making this an ineffective form of birth control.

Remember: Condoms don't last forever. Condoms are made of silicone or latex, and can expire just like food! Expired condoms are more likely to break or form holes than new condoms. Don't use the old condom you found on your sibling's nightstand. Expired condoms are a huge cause of teen pregnancy.

Girl, Protect Yourself

Sex is exciting and new. It's a great way to explore your body and express your love to a partner.

But while sex is fun, STDs and unplanned pregnancy are not.

Luckily, there are many ways to protect yourself and your partner from dangerous diseases.

This chapter covered some heavy stuff, but I don't want you to be scared. Instead of feeling anxious, use what you've learned about safe sex to make educated decisions about your body.

There's nothing embarrassing about having sex or discussing contraception. There are many resources available to you if you find yourself in a sticky situation. You deserve to know the facts.

Learning about safe sex, regardless of your choice to engage in it or not, is key to being a well-informed adult.

Period Pennings

Hopefully, you learned a lot from this chapter. We covered safe sex, pregnancy, contraception, and the value of protecting yourself.

Fill in the blanks to the questions provided below. Don't be afraid to be honest. No one has to read what you've written but you. Reflect on what you've learned and use these questions to understand what you know and how you can use the information I provided.

- I want to engage in sexual activity so I plan to do _____, _____, and _____ to protect myself.
- I want to learn more about trying _____ to protect myself

against pregnancy.

- I'm nervous about trying _____ because of _____, _____, and _____.
- This chapter taught me that _____ is important to becoming an informed adult.
- Before reading, I thought _____ and _____ were effective forms of contraception. I learned they aren't because of _____.

Conclusion: Moving Into The Beyond

I want you to think about the misconceptions you held true before reading this book. How do you feel now?

Hopefully, more at ease.

In this book, we discussed the positives of periods, including how to take care of your body while on your period and how they celebrate the process in many other cultures. We looked at chronic sleepiness and how it relates to your environment and how good nutrition simply doesn't go out of style.

You've learned how to live boldly and the value of embracing your body. There are always things we'd like to change; loving your body involves looking at the bird's-eye image, not the photo you see in front of you.

We learned about mental health and the warning signs, discovering gender identity, and the value of safe sex. Expression and identity are completely different; express yourself in a way that makes you feel comfy and confident.

You learned about teen pregnancy and the complications that may arise. Remember, having the knowledge necessary to make educated decisions is important, regardless of your choice to or not to engage in sex.

Growing up isn't easy. Your breast won't grow overnight, your pants will fit differently, and you might find yourself struggling to keep up with our society's hustle culture.

Believe me, I've been there.

And while there's no magic wand that will erase the difficulties of growing up, there are ways you can cope with the change head-on.

Take me, for example. I fell into the trap of doing what was expected of me. I felt the need to raise the bar again and again, only to find myself dissatisfied. So, I examined my body closely — I squeezed my nose in the mirror, felt ashamed when stepping on scales, and felt utterly alone during conversations about sexuality.

My teenage years were difficult and, in many ways, I'm still healing and learning from the process.

But you don't have to face the struggles I did; use the tools and information provided in this book.

With a little self-reflection and self-care, you too can be your own grown-up girl boss.

You are entering a new phase of your life where you begin to prepare for adulthood. You have the chance to shape your life according to your ambitions and desires. If you want to become a teacher, you can pursue that path by attending seminars, taking advantage of internships, and working hard in school. If you'd like to become a social worker, you can do a job shadow and decide you love helping others.

You might find your path changes over time. Mine certainly did! I started high school wanting to be a nurse and, when I graduated, I wanted to be a neonatal surgeon. It didn't work out either way, and that's alright!

This is where you start; this is the time you begin your journey as a lady.

If that seems a little too daunting, then you can start with being... Ladyish.

If this book helped you discover yourself and explore new avenues of being a teenager, leave a review and let's get in touch.

No one has to go through this process alone.

Remember, you can be ladyish however it suits you.

Thank you for your purchase! If you are happy with your book, Ladyish, please take a minute to review it here.

Ladyish:

https://www.amazon.com/review/create-review/?asin=B0 BJMVHS6M

References

Abma, J., & Martinez, G. (2019, May 24). *Over half of U.S. teens have had sexual intercourse by age 18, new report shows.* Www.cdc.gov. https://www.cdc.gov/nchs/pressroom/nchs_press_releases/2017/201706_NSFG.htm#:~:text=The%20report%20documented%20the%20following

Adhikari, S. (2019, September 29). *Teenage pregnancy: causes, effects and preventive measures.* Public Health Notes. https://www.publichealthnotes.com/teenage-pregnancy-causes-effects-and-preventive-measures/

Allure. (2018). *Girls ages 6-18 talk about body image | Allure.* In YouTube. https://www.youtube.com/watch?v=5mP5RveA_tk

American Academy of Pediatrics. (2019). *A teenager's nutritional needs.* HealthyChildren.org. https://www.healthychildren.org/English/ages-stages/teen/nutrition/Pages/A-Teenagers-Nutritional-Needs.aspx

Aquino, L. (2020, October 24). *5 menstrual rituals around the world | The Fornix | Flex.* The Fornix | Flex®. https://blog.flexfits.com/menstrual-rituals-around-the-world/Artdaily. (n.d.).

Are there birth control shot side effects? (n.d.). Www.plannedparenthood.org. https://www.plannedparenthood.org/learn/birth-control/birth-control-shot/birth-control-shot-side-effects

Behring, S. (2021, September 29). *What age do girls get their period?* Healthline. https://www.healthline.com/health/wom ens-health/what-age-do-girls-get-their-period#what-it-mea ns

Better Health Channel. (2018, November 5). *Teenagers and sleep.* Vic.gov.au; Better health channel. https://www.betterhe alth.vic.gov.au/health/healthyliving/teenagers-and-sleep

Bhandanker, K. (2017, November 13). *The effects of sexual harassment on teens.* The Swaddle. https://theswaddle.com/ effects-of-sexual-harassment-on-teens/

Birth control pill: contraception, the pill, effectiveness, types. (2020, July 21). Cleveland Clinic. https://my.clevelandclini c.org/health/drugs/3977-birth-control-the-pill#:~:text=Hor mones%20in%20birth%20control%20pills

Bradley University. (n.d.). *Bradley University: Disability & body image.* Www.bradley.edu. https://www.bradley.edu/sites /bodyproject/disability/body/

Brazier, Y. (2020, October 11). *Body image: What is it and how can I improve it?* Www.medicalnewstoday.com. https://www. medicalnewstoday.com/articles/249190

Bridges, F. (2017, July 21). *10 ways to build confidence.* Forbes. https://www.forbes.com/sites/francesbridges/2017/07/21/1 0-ways-to-build-confidence/?sh=5b0b060f3c59

Brink, S. (2019). *NPR choice page.* Npr.org. https://www.np r.org/sections/goatsandsoda/2015/08/11/431605131/attent ion-trump-some-cultures-treat-menstruation-with-respect

Cherry, K. (2020, November 21). *Why body positivity is important.* Verywell Mind. https://www.verywellmind.com/ what-is-body-positivity-4773402

Columbia Health Staff. (n.d.). *Body image concerns* | Columbia Health. Www.health.columbia.edu. https://www.health.colu

mbia.edu/content/body-image-concerns

Damour, L. (2022). *Speaking of psychology: Anxiety and teen girls.* Apa.org. https://www.apa.org/news/podcasts/speaking-of-psychology/anxiety-teen-girls

11 facts about sexual health in teens in the US. (2015). DoSomething.org. https://www.dosomething.org/us/facts/11-facts-about-sexual-health-teens-us

Gavin, M. (2018, May). *Breasts and bras (for kids)* - Nemours KidsHealth. Kidshealth.org. https://kidshealth.org/en/kids/breasts-bras.html

Gavin, M. (2019). *How much sleep do I need? (for teens)* - KidsHealth. Kidshealth.org. https://kidshealth.org/en/teens/how-much-sleep.html

Gender identity. (2021, March). Www.caringforkids.cps.ca. https://caringforkids.cps.ca/handouts/behavior-and-development/gender-identity

Gender identity, gender diversity and gender dysphoria: children and teenagers. (2021, March 15). Raising Children Network. https://raisingchildren.net.au/pre-teens/development/pre-teens-gender-diversity-and-gender-dysphoria/gender-identity

Glamour. (2020). *100 years of teen girls fashion | Glamour.* YouTube. https://youtu.be/sORunvibOYY

Griffin, L. (2020, October 5). *The effect of fashion on teenage mental health.* Mindless Mag. https://www.mindlessmag.com/post/the-effect-of-fashion-on-teenage-mental-health

Harvey, L. (n.d.). *Discussing your sexuality with your family and friends.* Www.bupa.com. https://www.bupa.com/news/stories-and-insights/2020/discussing-sexuality-with-family-and-friends

Hurley, K. (2017). *Anxiety in teens: The hidden signs of*

teen anixety you need to know. PsyCom.net - Mental Health Treatment Resource since 1986. https://www.psycom.net/hidden-signs-teen-anxiety/

Is your teen prepared for safe sex? (2017). Mayo Clinic. https://www.mayoclinic.org/healthy-lifestyle/sexual-health/in-depth/teens-and-sex/art-20045927

John Muir Health. (2019). *Nutrition for teens.* Johnmuirhealth.com. https://www.johnmuirhealth.com/health-education/health-wellness/childrens-health/nutrition-teens.html

Jones, E. (2016, September 15). *7 reasons getting your period is in fact GREAT.* Cosmopolitan. https://www.cosmopolitan.com/uk/body/health/a45944/why-your-period-actually-great/

Klein, Y. (2019, December 10). *Why is my teen always so tired? Do they have depression?* Evolve Treatment Centers. https://evolvetreatment.com/blog/teen-tired-fatigue-depression/

Marner, K. (2013, January 30). *When your daughter's worry is something more.* ADDitude. https://www.additudemag.com/what-anxiety-feels-like-for-teen-girls/

Mayo Clinic Staff. (2018). *Healthy body image: Tips for guiding girls.* Mayo Clinic. https://www.mayoclinic.org/healthy-lifestyle/tween-and-teen-health/in-depth/healthy-body-image/art-20044668

McQuenzie, L. (2020, May 29). *How do fashion trends affect teens?* Catwalk Yourself. http://www.catwalkyourself.com/fashion-news/how-do-fashion-trends-affect-teens/

National Eating Disorders Collaboration. (2021). *Body image.* Nedc.com.au. https://nedc.com.au/eating-disorders/eating-disorders-explained/body-image/

Nazario, B. (2021, February 10). *Safe sex mistakes to avoid.*

WebMD. https://www.webmd.com/sex/ss/slideshow-safe-se
x-mistakes-to-avoid

Nelson, E. (2021, March 12). *Am I next? Teenage girls and sexual harassment.* Healthconnected. https://www.health-co
nnected.org/post/am-i-next-teenage-girls-and-sexual-haras
sment

Olsson, R. (2020, August 23). *Is your daughter ready for a training bra?* | Banner Health. Www.bannerhealth.com. https://www.bannerhealth.com/healthcareblog/advise-me/
is-daughter-ready-for-a-training-bra

One-third of teenage girls sexually harassed online. (2017, December 6). BBC News. https://www.bbc.com/news/tec
hnology-42238118

Owen, C., & Pike, N. (2022, July 1). *How to measure for a bra that won't sabotage your day.* Vogue. https://www.vogue.com/
article/how-to-measure-for-a-bra

Pacheco, D. (2020, October 27). *Physical health and sleep: How are they connected?* Sleep Foundation. https://www.sleepfoun
dation.org/physical-health

Paul, B. (2020, December 3). *Patient education: Adolescent sexuality (beyond the basics)* UpToDate. Www.uptodate.com. https://www.uptodate.com/contents/adolescent-sexuality-b
eyond-the-basics

Peri, C. (2009, December 30). *How to stay awake naturally.* WebMD; WebMD. https://www.webmd.com/sleep-disorders
/features/natural-tips-sleepiness

Philadelphia, T. C. H. of. (2014, August 23). *Premenstrual syndrome (PMS).* Www.chop.edu. https://www.chop.edu/cond
itions-diseases/premenstrual-syndrome-pms

Pietro, S. (2016, January 15). *Mood disorders and teenage girls.* Child Mind Institute; Child Mind Institute. https://childmind.

org/article/mood-disorders-and-teenage-girls/

Qasim, A. (2019, October 18). *How do people around the world celebrate periods?* ActionAid UK. https://www.actionaid.org.uk /blog/news/2019/10/18/how-do-people-around-the-world-celebrate-periods

Raising Children. (2017, February 2). *Body image: Pre-teens and teenagers.* Raisingchildren.net.au. https://raisingchildren .net.au/pre-teens/healthy-lifestyle/body-image/body-image-teens

Sandesh, A. (2019, September 29). *Teenage pregnancy: Causes, effects and preventive measures.* Public Health Notes. https://ww w.publichealthnotes.com/teenage-pregnancy-causes-effects-and-preventive-measures/

Sclamberg, A. (2012, February 23). *What does food have to do with fashion?* HuffPost. https://www.huffpost.com/entry/eat-well_b_1288256

Sexual harassment: What kids and teens can do. (n.d.). Www.stompoutbullying.org. https://www.stompoutbullyi ng.org/teen-sexual-harassment-what-to-do

Shipman, C., Kay, K., & Ellyn, J. (2018, September 20). *How puberty kills girls' confidence.* The Atlantic. https://www.theatla ntic.com/family/archive/2018/09/puberty-girls-confidence/ 563804/

Singh, R. S. (2019, December 26). *Types of bras - 26 bra styles every women should know about* | Clovia. Clovia Blog. https://w ww.clovia.com/blog/21-types-of-bras-you-should-know-ab out/

Sleep and teens - UCLA Sleep Disorders Center - Los Angeles, CA. (n.d.). Www.uclahealth.org. https://www.uclahealth.org/ sleepcenter/sleep-and-teens#:~:text=There%20is%20a%20sh ift%20in

Smith, M., Robinson, L., & Segal, J. (2019, January 3). *Depression treatment.* HelpGuide.org. https://www.helpguide.org/articles/depression/depression-treatment.htm

Smith, M., Robinson, L., Segal, J., & Reid, S. (2018, December 20). *Parents guide to teen depression.* HelpGuide.org. https://www.helpguide.org/articles/depression/parents-guide-to-teen-depression.htmStanborough, R. (2020, November 25). *Negative body image: Definition, causes, symptoms, treatment.* Healthline. https://www.healthline.com/health/negative-body-image#definition

Starting your periods. (2018, April 9). Nhs.uk. https://www.nhs.uk/conditions/periods/starting-periods/#:~:text=Your%20periods%20will%20start%20when

Suni, E. (2020, October 23). How Sleep Works: Understanding the Science of Sleep. Sleep Foundation. https://www.sleepfoundation.org/how-sleep-works

Teen Mental Health: Facts & Statistics. (2018). Principles Academy for Adolescent Wellness. https://adolescentwellnessacademy.com/teen-mental-health-facts-statistics/

Teen Sexual Health. (n.d.). Medlineplus.gov. https://medlineplus.gov/teensexualhealth.html

Teenage sexuality. (2021, April 27). Raising Children Network. https://raisingchildren.net.au/pre-teens/development/puberty-sexual-development/teenage-sexuality

The impact of fashion trends on teenagers. Artdaily.cc. https://artdaily.cc/news/106451/The-Impact-of-Fashion-Trends-on-Teenagers#.Yt7OjxPMKrd

Trew, G. (2011). Pop Culture And Sexuality. The Missing Slate. http://journal.themissingslate.com/article/pop-culture-sexuality/

What causes sexual orientation? (n.d.). Www.plannedparenthood.org. https://www.plannedparenthood.org/learn/sexual-orientation/sexual-orientation/what-causes-sexual-orientation

What You Can Do to Stop Sexual Harassment | SHARE Title IX. (n.d.). Share.stanford.edu. https://share.stanford.edu/get-informed/stanford-resources/what-sexual-harassment/what-you-can-do-stop-sexual-harassment

Worley, W. (2016, March 11). Women officially need more sleep than men. The Independent. https://www.independent.co.uk/life-style/health-and-families/health-news/women-need-more-sleep-because-of-their-complex-brains-research-suggests-a6925266.html

Worried about your gender identity? Advice for teenagers. (2022, March 2). Nhs.uk. https://www.nhs.uk/live-well/trans-teenager/

Your First Period – Your Period. (n.d.). Www.yourperiod.ca. https://www.yourperiod.ca/normal-periods/your-first-period/Your teen's sexual orientation. (n.d.). Caringforkids.cps.ca. https://caringforkids.cps.ca/handouts/preteens-and-teens/teens_sexual_orientation

www.ingramcontent.com/pod-product-compliance
Lightning Source LLC
Chambersburg PA
CBHW052021030426

42335CB00026B/3240